7/00

Living with Genetic Disorder

Living with Genetic Disorder

The Impact of Neurofibromatosis 1

JOAN ABLON

AUBURN HOUSE
Westport, Connecticut • London

Library of Congress Cataloging-in-Publication Data

Ablon, Joan.
    Living with genetic disorder : the impact of neurofibromatosis 1 /
Joan Ablon.
      p. cm.
    Includes bibliographical references and index.
    ISBN 0–86569–287–4 (alk. paper)
    1. Neurofibromatosis—Social aspects. 2. Neurofibromatosis—
Psychological aspects. I. Title.
    [DNLM: 1. Neurofibromatosis 1 Personal Narratives. QZ 380 A152L
1999]
    RC280.N4A25 1999
    362.1′9699383—dc21
    DNLM/DLC
    for Library of Congress   99–11894

British Library Cataloguing in Publication Data is available.

Library of Congress Catalog Card Number: 99–11894
ISBN: 0–86569–287–4

First published in 1999

Auburn House, 88 Post Road West, Westport, CT 06881
An imprint of Greenwood Publishing Group, Inc.
www.greenwood.com

Printed in the United States of America

The paper used in this book complies with the
Permanent Paper Standard issued by the National
Information Standards Organization (Z39.48–1984).

10 9 8 7 6 5 4 3 2 1

Copyright Acknowledgments

The author and publisher gratefully acknowledge permission to quote from the following:

Portions of Chapter 9 are reprinted from *Social Science and Medicine*, Vol. 42, No. 1, Joan Ablon, Gender Response to Neurofibromatosis 1, pp. 99–109, copyright 1996, with permission from Elsevier Science.

Portions of Chapter 11 are reprinted from *Social Science and Medicine*, Vol. 40, No. 11, Joan Ablon, "The Elephant Man" as "Self" and "Other": The Psycho-social Costs of a Misdiagnosis, pp. 1481–1489, copyright 1995, with permission from Elsevier Science.

Portions of Chapter 12 appeared in Joan Ablon, Coping with Visible and Invisible Stigma: Neurofibromatosis 1, pp. 45–49. In *Accessing the Issues: Current Research in Disability Studies*, edited by Elaine Makas, Beth Haller, and Tanis Doe. Lewiston, ME: Society for Disability Studies and the Edmund S. Muskie Institute of Public Affairs, 1998. Reprinted with permission.

Selected passages in this volume appeared in Joan Ablon, Intangibles: The Psychologic Implications of Uncertainty, Diagnosis, Chronicity, and Prognosis in NF. In *Psychosocial Aspects of the Neurofibromatoses: Impact on the Individual, Impact on the Family*. Jane Novak Pugh Conference Series, Volume 3, 1992. New York: National Neurofibromatosis Foundation, Inc. Reprinted with permission.

Contents

Preface

It is estimated that thirteen million persons in our society are affected by genetic conditions that carry with them significant risks for physical or mental problems. Yet, the American public has little understanding of genetic disorders or of the issues faced by those who experience and carry them. Neurofibromatosis 1 (NF1), is a relatively common and complex neurological genetic disorder that affects as many as 100,000 persons in our society. However, little is known about this condition by the general public or even by many health care professionals. NF1 enjoyed a brief window of notoriety when it was mistakenly related to "The Elephant Man's Disease" and as such was highly popularized through the media. Many persons whose experiences are described here spent their formative or middle years in the frightening shadow of The Elephant Man. Through examining the complexities of this one condition, NF1, and some of its many consequences for affected individuals, one can gain an understanding of the parameters of living with other genetic conditions and the significance of genetic factors in the daily life of affected persons.

At the time of this writing there is no book that health care or social service providers or affected persons and their families can read to learn about the personal issues and concerns that many affected individuals with NF1 and other conditions are confronted with in the course of their lives. Because of the unpredictability of the condition, people with NF1 often feel their problems are unique. The few persons with NF1 they may have seen on television talk shows tend to be a severely and visibly affected but nonrepresentative sample of those with the condition.

My mission in this volume is to recount many shared personal and family experiences and examine the meanings of these for fifty-four persons who opened their lives to me. In most cases they had never before discussed these issues with another person. Despite the fact that NF1 may be manifested through many diverse symptoms, resulting in affected persons seeing a wide variety of health care professionals, most participants had little opportunity to share with professionals the personal issues of NF1 that had contributed significantly to the social and economic dimensions of their lives.

I am very appreciative of the support of the National Science Foundation (grant no. BN58819633) and an Academic Senate Research Grant from the University of California, San Francisco, which enabled me to carry out the field research on which this volume is based. I am grateful to Priscila Ednalgan, Kerry Lombardi, Elizabeth Steward, Terry Higgins, and Leslie Marcotte, who patiently typed many thousands of pages of transcripts and manuscripts; Paul Preston, who painstakingly coded the transcripts and field notes; Loreen Myerson, who ably assisted in the technical preparation; and Brooke Brown who helped with shortening the manuscript. I am greatly indebted to John C. Carey, M.D. and Susan M. Huson, M.D., for their ongoing enthusiastic support for this work and for generously sharing their great clinical knowledge of NF1 by reading a preliminary draft of the manuscript and offering numerous constructive and very helpful criticisms and suggestions. My thanks also go to Joan O. Weiss, Gay Becker, Renée Moore, Nora Bruemmer, Donna Warner, and the participant in this study whom I have called "Rachel," all of whom read and critiqued preliminary drafts. Friends Jean Pumphrey, Marilyn Leigh, and Gertrude Laney heroically encouraged my research efforts through the years of carrying out and writing up this study.

I am greatly appreciative of the ready assistance of the coordinators of the northern California support groups sponsored by the National Neurofibromatosis Foundation, Inc. and the California Neurofibromatosis Network. All of these coordinators, Nora Bruemmer, Marcia and Steve Ceccato, Dorothy Goldberg, Suzie McOmber, and Renée Moore and their families were helpful at every turn and graciously opened their meetings and their homes to me and allowed me to discuss my research plans, insights, and concerns with them and offered very helpful advice over the years of this study. The directors of the Genetics Departments of two major metropolitan hospitals contacted patients with information about my research. Judy Derstine was particularly helpful in locating NF1 patients for notification. The process of recruitment and follow-up of participants would have been much more difficult without the consistent support of all of these persons.

The participants in this study generously shared their life experiences and their perspectives on the ways that NF1 had touched their lives, hopes, and dreams. My intention with this volume is to facilitate and extend their remarkable sharing to others with NF1 and their families, to health care and social service professionals who work with them, and to the vast number of persons who live with the multiplicity of genetic disorders in our society.

1

Introduction

ROBBIE

I can deal with the surgeries and the threat of deafening, of blindness and paralysis—that's one thing. But, and it may seem vain, it's the disfigurement that bothers me. Society-wise, that is the most inhibiting thing. If I have surgery once or twice every few years people don't shun me for that. But if you look like you have some horrible skin condition, people just can really be cruel. I've had this fantasy—if I could just have twenty-four hours where I didn't have NF. Just to feel what it's like! Even if no one else could see me, and I just saw myself! It's a strange fantasy. Just to know what I would look like without it! And I try not to think how different my life would be if I hadn't had this. I try not to go on about "what if," because if I do that, I take away from my precious time now.

I sat in Robbie's apartment and watched this sensitive and solemn thirty-four-year-old man talk about his neurofibromatosis 1 (NF1) condition. His most poignant statements dealt with his inability to find a companion in life. He felt that his many bodily lesions had precluded a successful bid for relationships. He was extremely thin, with a long face, large brown eyes and a thatch of brown hair. When I came in, he positioned me into a big easy chair and he sat on the sofa facing me so that I was on his left side. I wondered if this was purposeful, because had I been on his right side I would be looking squarely at dozens, perhaps hundreds, of neurofibromas on his neck and face and also a large chasm where a tumor "half as big as [his] fist" had been removed near his ear.

The NF has been a massive determining factor on my whole life. I can't think of any period of my life where NF hasn't had a major effect. Even when I wasn't consciously aware of it for a time, it was a major contributing factor as to what I did or didn't do.

Robbie's apartment was small with a green shag carpet and tasteful furniture. Many religious pictures adorned the walls. The apartment was immaculate.

Robbie told me how members of his Catholic Church group had brought him food and taken him to the doctor during the past year of intensive postoperative treatment and recuperation following severe back surgery. He was to return to work part time the next day and was elated at the prospect of productive employment again and regaining the companionship of his workmates.

The symptoms Robbie relayed to me typified the major problems that confront persons with NF1: externally visible tumors that Robbie felt drastically affected his social life, and internal ones that seriously threatened his health and mobility. Learning disabilities beleaguered his educational and employment career.

SARAH

I told the doctor that having scars on my face and being disfigured has caused problems for me, and that repetitive surgeries have held me back. His response was, "Well, that's sociological, not medical." But if it were not for the medical, I would not incur these sociological problems.

I sat in a fast food restaurant booth with Sarah, a slender, black-haired thirty-eight-year-old woman facially marked by eleven past surgeries to remove tumors in her mouth and around her nose and eyes. In our numerous meetings over three years she had chronicled a difficult life—early sexual abuse by a family member, merciless teasing by schoolmates because of her unusual appearance and learning disabilities, teenage rape, and two abusive husbands. Sarah had called to tell me she was leaving Scott, her current husband, and she wished to talk about her options. There were few. Said Sarah:

Disabled women are not the women who tend to marry. Or, maybe they marry very often.

What do you mean?

Since people with disfigurements have low self-esteem, people like me get the message, "You're not okay; you're not pretty; you better take anything that comes along. You better just snap 'im up and count yourself lucky." I think I basically did that. I took that on and assumed that if I meet a man and he's not overtly nasty, and he doesn't overtly abuse me right away, he must be okay. And so by marrying often, I mean making repeated mistakes, and getting involved with relationships, running from one relationship to another. I haven't exactly done that. This is my second marriage, but it's not working out. And I certainly see a lot of the old patterns of my first marriage resurfacing.

Sarah had stayed with Scott in their chaotic household because she did not have the money to leave. Her minimum-wage job would not support her and her child (also affected by NF1) by a first marriage. The available welfare services and benefits offered no hope of a better standard of living without Scott and she needed either the support of another wage earner or disability benefits, which had been refused her, to help with upcoming surgery. She had already postponed this surgery numerous times, thereby threatening a positive surgical outcome. Within a few weeks Sarah did leave Scott, and she and her daughter were essentially homeless. They were staying with a friend the last time I saw her, but she had been given the warning that she would have to leave. The planned surgery went by the board.

Sarah's problems represented many of the experiences that women with physical or cognitive differences may encounter in American society. Sarah was able to articulate and analyze the issues she grappled with unusually well because of many hours of individual psychotherapy and group sessions at an abused women's shelter. Nonetheless, a successful escape from her lifelong cycle of abuse and poverty eluded her.

The diverse and complex problems of Robbie and Sarah exemplify but a few of the many consequences of NF1 for the lives of the persons described in this volume. From 1987 to 1995 I interviewed fifty-four NF1-affected adults and followed the lives of many of these over an eight-year period. I also interviewed eighteen families wherein there was an affected child of unaffected adults, that is, a mutation or "sporadic" case. This volume reports specifically on the lived experiences of affected adults. Becoming familiar with the seemingly enormous range of possible symptoms of NF1 was a sobering and complex educational experience. I marveled at the coping capacities of the persons that I interviewed. Most of these dealt not only with the immediate material features of NF1 but also the life consequences of serious learning disabilities and the uncertainty and insecurities spawned by their knowledge of the possibility of progression of physical symptoms. Societal stigma awaited them at every turn, and the specter of "The Elephant Man," long misdiagnosed as having NF1, haunted many of them from their teenage years. Was this the future they must look forward to? Typically these affected persons had never before spoken with another about their experiences or concerns. Their sharing imbued in me a very special mandate to make known their stories and experiences. What insights into the human condition and the possibilities of resilience did we learn from the compelling story of The Elephant Man? What insights are possible from gaining an understanding of the hopes, fears, and dreams of this population, so long associated with that tragic figure?

NEUROFIBROMATOSIS

The term *neurofibromatosis* ordinarily refers to two genetic disorders: neurofibromatosis 1, historically called von Recklinghausen Disease, the focus of this study, and neurofibromatosis 2, bilateral acoustic neurofibromatosis, a condition much less common and potentially more serious than neurofibromatosis 1. These two conditions were sometimes confounded for many years, but were more clearly separated in the mid-1970s. NF1 is considered to be a common disorder, occurring in one in 4,000 births, with 100,000 people in the United States estimated to have the condition. One-half of all cases represent new (de novo) mutations of the NF1 gene, and NF1 is one of the most common spontaneous mutations occurring in humans. In fact, NF1 affects more individuals than Tay-Sachs disease, muscular dystrophy, and Huntington's Chorea combined. NF1 is an autosomal dominant condition, occurring equally across gender, racial, ethnic, and national boundaries. An affected parent has a 50 percent chance in every birth of passing on the condition. The issues of decision making around childbearing are frequently complex and painful ones for prospective parents. Some of these issues will be discussed in Chapter 8.

The most common manifestations of NF1 are cafe-au-lait spots (darkened patches on the skin commonly called "birth marks." Some 10 percent of the general population have these marks but in smaller numbers and size than is common in NF1). The other most common defining features are neurofibromas or smallish tumors on the skin, and skin fold freckling. Neurofibromas develop in and along nerves and nerve sheaths, which are present all through the body. Neurofibromas ordinarily appear after adolescence and may increase in number throughout the life span. Many women experience a burgeoning of neurofibromas during or following pregnancy. Most of the persons that I interviewed had at least a slight sprinkling of neurofibromas on the torso and often had a significant number of them. The spread of these to the neck, face, and arms spells the public manifestation of NF1. External neurofibromas may be cosmetically disfiguring and associated with considerable stigma for an affected person. Internal neurofibromas may impinge on vital organs, impede mobility, and be potentially malignant.

Learning disorders also are commonly associated with NF1 and are reported in some studies to plague up to 50 percent of affected persons. Learning disorders are profiled as a major destructive factor in the lives of the subjects described in this volume. When these adult subjects were in school, learning disorders typically were not recognized. Subjects often were called "dumb" or "lazy," and the negative effects of this labeling have followed many of them to the present day. Many children with learning disabilities today are identified early in their school experience and are given special school and class placements and sometimes see a variety of specialists.

The manifestations of NF1 are of considerable variety, and the rate of progression of the disorder can vary dramatically in different individuals even within the same family. NF1's most damaging psychological feature is its unpredictability.

It should be noted that persons who come for medical services and to support groups may represent the more serious end of an unknown spectrum. Thus available figures on the condition are disproportionately weighted toward severity and may represent those with moderate or severe problems. Clinicians often state that most persons with NF1 have few or no medical problems, and in fact, some geneticists have commented that possibly as many as half of the persons who have NF1 never know of its existence in their lifetime. While clinicians tend to believe that most persons with NF1 are not and will not be severely affected, it should be noted that clinical assessments ordinarily do not factor in the *psychosocial impact* of symp-

toms such as external neurofibromas, which may or may not be clinically threatening, yet might influence not only experiences of daily life, but also major expectations, opportunities, and decisions throughout the life course. Fuller descriptions
of NF1, its symptoms, and treatment are presented in Appendix I. For detail on all
aspects of NF1 and its management, the reader is directed to Rubenstein and Korf
(1990), Riccardi (1992), Huson and Hughes (1994), Gutmann et al. (1997), and
Upadhyaya and Cooper (1998).

Enormous advances in scientific knowledge about the cause of NF1 have
occurred in the past decade. The gene for NF1, located on chromosome 17, and the
protein it produces, neurofibromin, were identified in 1990. The NF1 gene is
thought to be a tumor suppressor gene, which also makes it of interest to cancer
researchers. The gene is a large one and unraveling its many mysteries may be years
away.

HISTORY OF NF1

While researchers suggest that NF1 was identified in graphic portrayals even as
early as the second century, and written about in numerous works in the centuries
following, it was first described clearly by Friedrich Daniel von Recklinghausen in
1882, and thereafter was commonly called "von Recklinghausen Disease." NF1
was essentially unknown to the general public until it was related to "The Elephant
Man's Disease" through the publication of Ashley Montagu's book, *The Elephant
Man: A Study in Human Dignity*, in 1971. Montagu's book was centered on the
major essay of the British nineteenth-century surgeon Sir Frederick Treves' volume,
The Elephant Man and Other Reminiscences, published in 1923. Montagu presented Treves' vivid and moving twenty-five page account of Joseph Merrick, an
unfortunate young Englishman so grossly disfigured that he lived a miserable life
as a carnival attraction.

The hero of this story . . . lived just short of twenty-six years, most of them spent in a living
purgatory. Hideously deformed, malodorous, for the most part maltreated, constantly in pain,
lame, fed the merest scraps, exhibited as a grotesque monster at circuses, fairs, and wherever
else a penny might be turned, the object of constant expressions of horror and disgust.
(Montagu 1971:2)

In 1884 Treves brought Merrick to London Hospital where he lived for the next
four years until his death at age twenty-five. His courage and dignity deeply touched
many prominent persons of the day who visited him there.

Merrick's condition was diagnosed as NF1 early in this century and this
misdiagnosis existed until 1986 when his condition was rediagnosed as "Proteus
Syndrome," a much rarer and more serious disorder than NF1. However, the vivid
portrayal of Merrick's life on American stage, screen, and television parlayed the
designation of his condition into a household phrase, a metaphor for the grimmest
extreme of ugliness. The consequences of the diagnosis of The Elephant Man's

Disease as NF1 have been major for many of those persons with the condition and for the scientific quest to understand and find a cure for NF1. The Elephant Man phenomenon and its sequelae will be presented in more detail in Chapter 11.

GENETIC DISORDERS

Recent international attention to genetic structure and inheritance as a major determinant in our lives has come as a consequence of the Human Genome Project, the primary mission of which is to map, identify, and analyze the 100,000 genes operant in the human body. Since it began in 1988, the Human Genome Project has resulted in remarkable progress in laboratories around the world, aided by the high technology of molecular genetics (Collins and Fink 1995). Our newspapers daily announce new discoveries of the genes for both common and rare conditions. Up to this time public attention had been drawn episodically to the poignancy of such dramatic conditions as cystic fibrosis or the "Bubble Boy" syndrome. Much more familiar in life encounters is Down syndrome, a relatively common chromosomal disorder.

Collins has observed, "There are no perfect genetic specimens. All of us carry an estimated five to fifty significant genetic flaws" (Collins 1998). The medical, economic, social, and emotional consequences of genetic disorders are enormous. Genetic disorders constitute a major cause of morbidity and mortality in this country. A large proportion of both pediatric and adult hospital admissions are due to genetic disorders. Three percent of all pregnancies result in the birth of a child with a significant disorder that can cause serious disease or death. If late onset, multifactorial disorders, those resulting from a combination of genes, are included, 60 percent of all individuals are thought to have genetically influenced conditions (Wynbrandt and Ludman 1991).

Approximately 5,700 genetic disorders affecting humans have been identified, and some 300 are detectable through genetic testing (Bobinski 1996:80). Screening tests are currently available to determine if a person is a carrier of such conditions as sickle cell anemia, Tay-Sachs disease, and cystic fibrosis, and future tests will reveal susceptibility to many other disorders. Following the precise identification of genetic materials that contribute to problematic conditions, prevention and treatment are expected to follow. Genetic therapies and various modes of genetic engineering may be developed to correct, enhance, and "improve" on physical and mental characteristics.

The knowledge resulting from the mapping of the human genome holds enormous import for the individual. Bobinski (1996) predicts the Human Genome Project will lead to the "geneticization of much of what we currently think of as our health, talents, and personality" (1996:107). Jonsen (1996) has noted:

Today . . . [health] risks are written in abstract numbers that have but remote impact on the way in which persons see themselves; tomorrow these risks will be written on each one's genome, an indelible part of the self. . . . Just as my genetics are me, so my mutations and disease that they in some way effect, will be me. (Jonsen 1996:10)

Such knowledge may vitally affect a person's sense of identity, and may seriously influence a person's choices in reproduction—whether to have children, or if having conceived, after prenatal testing whether to keep a genetically affected fetus or abort. Some of these issues will be discussed in Chapter 8.

While the Human Genome Project holds the promise of revealing the mysteries of many of the diseases that have beleaguered millions of persons, there exist imminent dangers in the possibility of making knowledge that is so intrusive to individuals and families essentially available to the world. Approximately 3 to 5 percent of the annual appropriation for the Human Genome Project is earmarked to support educational and research efforts focused on the ethical, legal, and social implications of the work being carried out in molecular genetics. Considerable attention is being given to many highly complex issues attendant to the Human Genome Project, such as those of genetic testing, maintaining the confidentiality and privacy of medical and genetic information, and concerns about the use of information. When once known that an individual is at risk for a specific condition that person may be excluded from employment or health insurance (see chapters in Murray et al. 1996; Weir et al. 1994; Cranor 1994; Suzuki and Knudtson 1990).

Genetic disorders carry with them special symbolic burdens that may sorely exacerbate the attendant physical symptomatology. In the case of a familial disease both the passers and the receivers often experience dramatic emotions. While mutations carry their share of guilt by unknowing and thus non-"responsible" parents, the passing of a known heritable condition has the potential for causing tremendous psychological upheavals. The symbolic implications of the family line carrying a serious or dread condition may affect all family members negatively.

Geneticists have pointed up the importance of "natural history" research as a component of clinical care. Hall has emphasized the study of natural history for prevention, therapy, and elicitation of aetiology. She defines natural history as:

An account of all the consequences of that disorder, or as the study of the disease process with emphasis on the sequence of events and the effects of time. This includes age of onset, initial complaints, signs, symptoms, laboratory aids in diagnosis, order of onset of complications and manifestations, the effect of the condition on pregnancy, age of death, types and effectiveness of treatments, as well as the modifications that the treatments produce, psychosocial ramifications, and even the impact of ethnic background and environmental factors. (Hall 1988:434)

Little is known about the psychosocial casualties of the numerous genetic conditions. Individual and family adaptation to genetic disorders has remained the least researched area of the gamut of provocative issues in this field. The most immediate and direct mode of gaining the psychosocial dimension of the natural history is through the elicitation of life stories or personal narratives such as those that form the basis for this volume. Anthropologists have been at the forefront of the few published works that examine personal and lifestyle issues. For example, see Ablon 1984, 1988, 1992b; Boutté 1987, 1990; Myerson, 1995.

PERSONAL NARRATIVES

Narratives help us to understand the "illness" response of individuals and families to genetic disorder. Social scientists and some medical researchers have distinguished between the terms "illness" and "disease." Kleinman (1988) clarifies the use of these terms:

When I use the word illness . . . I shall mean something fundamentally different from what I mean when I write disease. By invoking the term illness, I mean to conjure up the innately human experience of symptoms and suffering. Illness refers to how the sick person and the members of the family or wider social network perceive, live with, and respond to symptoms and disability. . . . Illness problems are the principal difficulties that symptoms and disability create in our lives.

Disease is the problem from the practitioner's perspective. In the narrow biological terms of the biomedical model, this means that disease is reconfigured *only* as an alteration in biological structure or functioning. . . . Disease, however, is what the practitioner creates in the recasting of illness in terms of theories of disorder. Disease is what practitioners have been trained to see through the theoretical lenses of their particular form of practice. That is to say, the practitioner reconfigures the patient's and family's illness problems as narrow technical issues, disease problems. (Kleinman 1988:3–4, 4–5)

Researchers have used personal narratives as a rich resource for the understanding of illness experiences. Reflecting the inner world of experiences, personal narratives are documents that "provide a density of texture, a depth of personal meaning, and an insight into the experience of illness not readily available through other means" (Robinson 1990:1173).

The cultural context and state of professional and lay understandings about a condition are significant factors in shaping persons' remembrances and recounting of events. The image an affected person has of his/her illness and future is closely tied to their perceptions of their doctors', family's, friends', and society's views of their condition. For example Hyden states, "An important aspect of the act of formulating one's thoughts about an illness is the rhetorical devices which patients, family and friends and professionals use when defining the nature and gravity of an illness" (Hyden 1995:84). These rhetorical aspects are central to how the illness is experienced and dealt with by the bearer of the illness and their associates. The modes of discourse used by doctors and the media may frame the individual's attitudes toward his/her condition, their resolve for maintenance regimens, and their optimism or pessimism about their prognosis.

In the case of NF1 the flamboyance of the misdiagnosed Elephant Man's Disease and the image of the tragic figure of Joseph Merrick was very influential in the development of shame and depression in many persons with NF1. Likewise the florid rhetoric used by doctors who told patients and families that this "rare" and "terrible" disease could likely result in severe disability was an important factor in the development of negative mindsets of many subjects about their condition. Further, for many affected subjects the only cultural representation of this heretofore unknown condition was that of The Elephant Man, or one of the severely (and statistically unrepresentative) affected persons that have been showcased on television talk shows.

DISABILITY AND STIGMA

In coming to understand the lived experience of having NF1 it is useful to consider this experience within the concepts of *disability* and *stigma*.

Disability

Physical impairment has been characterized as a "human constant," but one whose definition and social consequences vary enormously by cultural setting and through time. Scheer and Groce, in presenting cross-cultural and historical perspectives on physical difference, define disability conditions to include "genetic disorders, chronic or infectious diseases that cause permanent impairments, and injuries that lead to lifetime impairments" (Scheer and Groce 1988:23–24). They suggest that social scientists and policymakers alike tend to overlook the constant presence of impairments in human societies. The World Health Organization initially estimated that approximately 10 percent of the world's population are physically or mentally impaired at any given time. These figures were later modified to 6 or 7 percent, resulting in a global figure of 245 million disabled persons (Helander, 1993). The ambiguity around these figures reflects issues surrounding inclusion or exclusion of varied conditions that may constitute "disability" around the world. While the concept of disability is a familiar one in our society, it is difficult to make cross-cultural generalizations about "disability" or "impairment" because in many cultures disability as a recognized category does not exist. For discussions of various cultural conceptions of disability see Whyte and Ingstad 1995.

In the United States many conditions typically are subsumed under the term "disability." Disability issues fall within the realms of the legal, social and economic. States LaPlante (1992):

Under the Americans with Disabilities Act of 1990 (ADA), a person with a disability is defined as one with "a physical or mental impairment that substantially limits one or more of the major life activities of such individual." [Major life activities include those such as walking, seeing, hearing, speaking, working, breathing, learning, caring for oneself.] . . . As defined by regulations implementing Section 504 of the Rehabilitation Act of 1973—the legal antecedent of the ADA—physical impairments include "any physiological disorder or condition, cosmetic disfigurement, or anatomical loss" . . . affecting the major body systems of the human organism. Mental impairments include "any mental or psychological disorder, such as mental retardation, organic brain syndrome, emotional or mental illness, and specific learning disabilities." . . . By the qualifying words "substantial" and "major life activity," the ADA definition intends to focus on significant limitations in human activities. (LaPlante 1992:1)

The 1990 National Health Interview Survey estimates that 22.9 million persons of all ages living in households in the United States are limited in major activity. An additional 10.9 million are estimated to have "nonmajor" activity limitations such as difficulty performing civic, church, and recreational activities (Adams and Benson 1991).

While most persons might envision disability as typified by a mobility-impaired person with spinal cord injury, numerous other disabilities have been recognized for economic assistance, special rehabilitation and education, and protection from discrimination. The clumping of such broadly diverse conditions as spinal cord injury and learning disabilities renders generalizations about "disability" and "disabled persons" as tentative or highly complicated at best. However most disabled persons, whatever their condition might be, are faced with significant social and attitudinal barriers as well as logistic ones that function to complicate their daily life experiences, humiliating them and frustrating their expectations and aspirations for a normal life. Stigma is a frequent accompaniment of disability.

A Redefinition of Disability. A major distinction must be made between the physical or functional impairment a person may have and the environmental barriers—logistic, social, economic, or political—in their life which often determine the problems they may experience. For example, in most cases the symptoms of NF1 described in this volume would not have caused as serious consequences for affected persons if learning disabilities had been appropriately attended to, if legal remedies for discrimination in education and employment had been in place and enforced, and if the cosmetic prescriptions of our society were not so rigid and all-encompassing.

Scholars in disabilities studies and disability rights advocates emphasize the above distinction and a sociocultural constructionist perspective on disability. *The locus of disability problems lies in the political, social, and economic systems that deny equal rights and opportunities to disabled persons, not in personal deficiencies of individuals.* Further, these problems may be better understood not as medical or welfare problems but as civil rights issues of prejudice toward an underprivileged minority. Hahn has observed, "the extent to which environmental modifications could ameliorate the functional constraints of a disability may eventually be determined by technology and by the limits of human imagination in designing a world adapted to the needs of everyone" (Hahn 1988:40). Persons with disabilities who have internalized this realization may proceed more positively and with more confidence and sense of control because the environment, by common effort, can and will be changed.

The causes and consequences of differing conditions that fit under the broad rubric of "disability" may vary dramatically, but persons with these conditions typically all confront varying degrees of stigma and resulting discrimination in our society. The diversity of physical and mental impairments may preclude a group consciousness or individual recognition of sharing a particular status or belonging to a category of persons. Indeed, as is true for persons with NF1, "disability is an individualized experience for most people" (Scotch 1988:161). Persons with disabilities often feel that they are the only ones with their special condition. The person with a disability usually grows up with and is surrounded by nondisabled family, friends, schoolmates, and workmates. Thus, a diversity of conditions and geographic dispersement tend to discourage the social and physical development of a community of disability. Likewise, Scotch has observed, "The social status of being disabled can create serious disincentives for many to identify themselves as disabled and act collectively on that basis. To be perceived as disabled is typically to be seen as helpless and incompetent, and many individuals with physical impairments seek to disassociate themselves from disability" (Scotch 1988:161).

I find useful Howe's (1964) concept of community as a *symbolic* community of interest, composed of persons who may be geographically dispersed and hence not known to one another but who share similar significant characteristics that create for them a "common destiny." In this sense the shared experiences and concerns of persons with disabilities have the potential to unite them for psychological support and political action.

A major coming together of persons with disabilities and those who live and work with them to form a disabilities rights movement achieved its major momentum during the 1970s and 1980s. Persons with disabilities stepped forward to achieve the same protection and rights under the law as had other underprivileged minorities in those years. Political activism has since resulted in laws that have made discrimination in education, employment, and access to public facilities illegal. The most far-reaching of these laws was the Americans with Disabilities Act of 1990.

While many persons with NF1 would not consider themselves to be "disabled," associating that term with mobility impairment, in reality some 75 percent of my sample would fit within the categories outlined in the ADA. Actual learning disabilities affected more than one-half of the persons. Others had serious mobility, mental health, or cosmetic issues that limited normal functioning in the tasks of daily living. Nine persons were primarily supported by disability benefits based on physical or emotional difficulties that precluded their being able to work. Others, while able-bodied, were so self-conscious about their numerous visible neurofibromas or other symptoms that they felt they could not work, date, marry, or in a few cases even shop or go to restaurants in their communities.

STIGMA

The impact of stigma, society's negative evaluation of particular features or behavior, was first significantly addressed by Goffman in his seminal work *Stigma: Notes on the Management of Spoiled Identity* (1963). Goffman stated:

Society establishes the means of categorizing persons and the complement of attributes felt to be ordinary and natural. . . . While the stranger is present before us, evidence can arise of his possessing an attribute that makes him different from others in the category of persons available for him to be, and of a less desirable kind—in the extreme, a person who is quite thoroughly bad, or dangerous, or weak. He is thus reduced in our minds from a whole and usual person to a tainted, discounted one. (Goffman 1963:5)

American values contain significant cosmetic and social prescriptions for "beauty," "ugliness," and "good health," which are systematically reinforced by portrayals in the media and through selection in social, economic, and political dimensions of life. Social success favors individualism, physical "health" and bodily "beauty," and athletic and vocational achievements. Negativity toward the physically or mentally different who may not be able to meet such prescriptions has been well documented by researchers (Goffman 1963; Safilios-Rothschild 1977; Eisenberg 1982; Eisenberg et al. 1982; Graham and Kligman 1985; Ablon 1984, 1988, 1995; Hatfield and Sprecher 1986; Livneh 1988; Yuker 1988; Grealy 1994). Zola (1985), in a review of media portrayals of disability, states that an important feature of media representations is the negative message concerning the way people with disabilities live out their lives. Zola notes that the relationships of the majority of persons portrayed as disabled were characterized as impotent and dependent.

Murphy (1990) offers a clear and vivid explication of the manner in which American values and the response of the American public to physical differences affect individuals and families who bear this mark:

there is a clear pattern in the United States, and in many other countries, of prejudice toward the disabled and debasement of their social status, which find their most extreme expressions in avoidance, fear, and outright hostility. . . . Whatever the physically impaired person may think of himself, he is attributed a negative identity by society, and much of his social life is a struggle against this imposed image. It is for this reason that we can say that stigmatization is less a by-product of disability than its substance. The greatest impediment to a person's taking full part in his society are not his physical flaws, but rather the tissue of myths, fears, and misunderstandings that society attaches to them. (Murphy 1990:112–113)

Persons with NF1 and other genetic disorders often find that they are stigmatized by the very fact that they are carrying a condition that is imprinted in their intrinsic genetic makeup. Quaid (1994) has noted:

Genetic information is widely viewed as saying something about who the person is at some fundamental, if unarticulated, level. In that sense, especially, people appear to feel stigmatized by exposure of their genetic information, and others might be more likely to stigmatize on that basis. In some cases, even medical professionals exhibit the tendency to treat proven genetic disorders in a manner different from the way they might treat other diseases, with predictable effects on individuals at risk. (Quaid 1994:6)

Hahn (1988) suggests that two chief elements in the attitudes of nondisabled toward disabled persons are *aesthetic* anxiety, a reaction to a physical difference that is regarded as unappealing or unattractive, and *existential* anxiety, a reaction that reflects fear by the nondisabled of the potential loss of their own functional capabilities. In this case an underlying thought might be, "There but for the grace of God go I." (Also Livneh 1988; Goffman 1963.) For examples of these elements, in many of the negative experiences around school and employment recounted by the subjects in this study of NF1, the apparent trigger would be subsumed within a functional limitations model. The inability of subjects to achieve a modal level of functional proficiency might cause others to fear that they might lose their own abilities. In contrast, social exclusion in dating would be based on an aesthetic anxiety, caused by perceived physical difference.

For persons with NF1, visible tumors, skeletal differences, learning disorders— virtually all of the large array of symptoms of NF1 may call forth the negative attention of classmates, workmates, the general public, and even family and friends. Children who are physically different in any way may be faced with a daily barrage of teasing and insults from playmates, schoolmates, and even teachers (Richman and Harper 1978; Ablon 1984, 1988; Breslau 1985; Wallander et al. 1989; Csapo 1991; Lansdown et al. 1991). Affected persons also may be stigmatized because of behaviors necessary for dealing with their condition such as absenteeism from school or work because of frequent doctors' visits. Adaptation to stigma and its consequences will be a chief area of examination in this volume.

THIS STUDY

What was the serendipitous path that brought me into the lives of persons with NF1? I came to this study from many years of working with individuals and families with another genetic condition—dwarfism (Ablon 1984, 1988). A chance encounter at a short stature symposium with a member of an NF support group whose husband and children had the condition then erroneously called "The Elephant Man's Disease" promised to open many windows on how individuals and families live with stigma, uncertainty, and many forms of disability as daily companions.

I interviewed fifty-four adults with NF1 concerning their life experiences and coping patterns around their condition. Subjects were recruited from three sources: (1) the population of persons attending three NF support groups in northern California sponsored by the National Neurofibromatosis Foundation, Inc. and the now historical California Neurofibromatosis Network; (2) those who had responded to notices placed in local mailing announcements of these two organizations; and (3) the caseloads of the genetics departments of two major metropolitan hospitals. I cannot state that the subjects reported on here are representative of all persons affected with NF1, since the exact constitution of the total universe of those persons is unknown. However, I believe that these subjects are a fair representation of many of the thousands who do attend support groups, who receive announcements but do not attend, and who come to hospital programs. It should be noted, however, that these sources may attract affected persons and families who are on the more severe end of the range of affected persons.

My interviewing took me into a very broad spectrum of residences and lifestyles over northern California. Subjects spanned enormous economic, social, and geographic differences—from modest homes and livelihoods in lumber mills and factories on the northern California coast to elaborate mansions and high technology offices of the San Francisco Bay area. I visited affluent suburban homes and inner-city ghetto apartments; from an evening with a wealthy matron complaining about her decorator's latest splurge, to a day with a young woman dressed in black leather clothing and chains who described the crack (cocaine)-related shootings on her block. One day I interviewed a Nicaraguan woman who recounted her undocumented crossing of the California border with a "coyote" (an illegal guide), and the next day a retired army officer in an exclusive senior village.

In most cases interviews were carried out in subjects' homes, and, in a few instances, in restaurants. Thirty-four subjects were interviewed one time; eleven subjects were interviewed twice; and nine others were interviewed three or more times—some five or six times over many years. Materials also were gathered at NF support group meetings and in telephone conversations. Subjects were generous in sharing with me their life experiences and attitudes toward their NF1. Interviews tended to last at least three hours and many were four or five hours or longer. Many persons stated that they had never before candidly talked to another person about their condition and the ways in which they perceived it had affected their lives.

Of the fifty-four affected adults who spoke with me, thirty-two were women and twenty-two were men. Fifteen had a parent with NF1. Twenty had affected children. Ten persons were members of ethnic minorities: five Latinos, three African Americans, one Chinese, and one Filipino. Ages of subjects ranged from nineteen to seventy at the time of the first interview.

Educational levels varied from completion of high school to enrollment in doctoral-level graduate courses. The occupations of subjects were so diverse that their number almost equaled the number of subjects. Vocations ranged through professionals, laborers, retirees, and persons living on temporary and permanent disability benefits. A more detailed listing of vocations appears in Chapter 6.

NF1 appears to be a great leveler in its affect on socioeconomic status. Many persons who were raised in middle class lifestyles are only able to maintain low-level or part-time jobs with few or no benefits and now live on the economic fringes of society. Often this is due to the diverse effects of learning disabilities and/or the necessity for frequent absences from work for surgeries or for doctors' appointments. Details of the sample are presented in Appendix II. Contextual information on the subjects who are most frequently quoted is presented in Appendix III.

SYMPTOMS, REACTIONS, AND CONSEQUENCES OF NF1

One of the most salient features of NF1 that became quickly apparent in the accounts of adult subjects was the remarkable heterogeneity of its presentations, both in clinical symptoms and their consequences. I was impressed by the subjective and highly variable nature of subjects' perceptions of the severity and import of their condition and of how it had influenced their lives. Any outsider's assessment of clinical severity or visibility cannot predict the affected person's own assessment of their condition, their anxieties about it, or the consequences of the condition for their lives.

These features make difficult the posing of broad generalizations about the impingement of NF1 on the lives of individuals and families and their psychological and practical modes of coping with their condition. The sample spanned individuals with one or two small lesions on their bodies to an amputee whose leg was removed because of a malignant NF1 tumor and a subject who was essentially totally paralysed following spinal surgery. Within this broad range were persons whose learning disabilities and physical symptoms rendered them unable to work, yet who stated they felt their lives would be little different without NF1. In contrast some very mildly affected persons were psychologically paralyzed because of their condition.

In an attempt to evaluate the importance of various factors in the adaptation of subjects to their condition I examined eight variables in relation to subjects' current lives. Some of these variables are intrinsic to the NF1 condition and others are elements of individual and family experiences. The variables are gender, age at diagnosis, presence of NF1 in a parent, socioeconomic status of parents, learning disorders, visibility, severity, and available support systems. The results of this examination will be discussed in the conclusion.

The following chapters will review the psychosocial literature on NF1 and then describe life experiences through subjects' own words. The chapters trace the life course beginning with diagnosis, and describe family response, school experiences, employment, dating and sexual behavior, marriage, childbearing, and medical experiences. A variety of issues such as living with uncertainty and stigma that were brought up time and time again in interviews are discussed. Varied dimensions of the impact of NF1 in subjects' lives are explored. Finally the significance of a number of factors that have contributed to positive adaptation to NF1 and to several other genetic disorders are discussed and suggestions for family and health care providers are presented.

2

Psychosocial Issues in Living with NF1

While there is a voluminous research literature on the clinical and physiological aspects of NF1, there exists but a handful of works that even refer to what Riccardi has called the *psychosocial burden* of NF1: "the obviously adverse effect of NF-1 on the emotional and social life of the patient" (Riccardi 1992:198). From his extensive clinical experience, psychological testing, and communications with hundreds of patients Riccardi states, "The vast majority of patients with NF-1 beyond early and middle childhood suffer some compromise of their overall psychosocial performance as a direct and/or indirect result of their disease" (Riccardi 1992:195). Further, Riccardi notes:

Any compromise of functions that are described in psychologic, emotional, and social terms must be considered as having three possible origins. First, there are factors that are *superimposed* merely as a function of the patient having a progressive, chronic, poorly understood disease, regardless of the details of the disorder's features. . . . Second, there are factors that represent *responses* to the patient's specific NF-1 features, such as cosmetic disfigurement or short stature. . . . These may be responses of the patient to himself or herself, either consciously or subconsciously, or responses of other persons or groups of persons, or both. Third, the *NF-1 mutation* may directly contribute to this type of compromise via primary disturbances of cell function within the brain itself. The information available to date does not allow a precise dissection of these factors in individual patients, though some broad generalizations can be made. (Riccardi 1992:195)

Riccardi discusses what he called "*dysmaturity*," various degrees of psychosocial immaturity manifested by excessive passivity and impoverished social performance, often in the context of symptoms of neuroses and hypochondriasis. Riccardi has identified this dysmaturity in patients from all socioeconomic strata and in all levels of severity; however, he notes that symptoms of this dysmaturity were more apparent in those patients in lower socioeconomic groups and in the categories of greatest severity (Riccardi 1992:196).

Messner and Neff Smith (1986) observed that an extensive review of the international literature suggested to them that the adaptations of individuals and families and implications of the provision of holistic care were only "superficially mentioned" in the hundreds of items of that literature. Messner, a nurse clinician and patient educator who also has NF2, has authored or coauthored most of the relatively few publications that address the personal and family coping and adaptation patterns of persons with NF (Messner 1986; Messner, Gardner, and Messner 1985; Messner, Messner, and Lewis 1985; Messner and Neff Smith 1986). Messner and colleagues wrote with passion, addressing the emotional adaptations that affected individuals make to the disorder, and they emphasize the manifestations of negative self-image that typically have resulted from societal insults around their condition. Because these authors wrote during the period in which The Elephant Man's Disease was misdiagnosed as NFI, they frequently allude to the profound impression made by the image of The Elephant Man on affected persons and their perception of their condition.

Messner and Neff Smith (1986) present their concept of "chromosomal coping," which involves the multilevel process of "(1) coping with NF and its accompanying medical, psychosocial and genetic sequelae; and (2) coping with life as it is affected by NF" (Messner and Neff Smith 1986:461). These authors point up the complexities of the psychological complications that may accompany NF1. They state:

Literally every tissue and organ of the body may be involved in NF by either tumors or associated entities; however, the disfiguring physical appearance generally creates the most psychological trauma. Patients with NF must cope with a multitude of losses—self-esteem, normal bodily function, key roles and role relationships, financial security, professional aspirations, unfulfilled reproductive drives, being a part of "normal" society, and, most importantly, loss of control. (Messner and Neff Smith 1986:461)

Addressing the issue of disfigurement, Messner (1986) observed:

The image of "The Elephant Man" continues to haunt many NF patients who are caught in the gap between a genetic error and the inability of medical science to rectify that error. Many individuals with NF must literally wear their diagnosis; patients even minimally affected by the disorder may adopt a negative self-concept, exceedingly disproportionate to the actual clinical manifestations. (Messner 1986:7)

Further, Messner, Gardner, and Messner (1985) noted:

Like the individual with anorexia nervosa who sees a blimp in the mirror, the NF patient may see "The Elephant Man" in his mirror, despite his actual physical appearance. This identity disorder intensifies social isolation, and attempts to make a manifestation less noticeable may literally consume the patient's energy. (Messner, Gardner, and Messner 1985:319)

Messner and Neff Smith state that practitioners throughout the literature consistently describe NF patients as generally being "creative, sensitive, unusually kind individuals, not embittered by their condition" (Messner and Neff Smith 986:462). For example, Trevisani et al. (1982) stated:

Patients afflicted also may suffer irreversible psychological scarring and are often looked upon by others as freakishly grotesque. However, considering their circumstances, they tend to be even-tempered and gentle people longing for acceptance. Most are not embittered by their affliction. (Trevisani et al. 1982:217)

Likewise, Marchac noted: "These patients are often very intelligent, are remarkably gentle and cooperative, and are willing to undergo multiple procedures" (Marchac 1984:540).

My own research findings offer a contrast to the perceptions of the latter clinicians about their patients, as will be discussed more fully in Chapter 15 and in the Conclusion. I found subjects to be often high-spirited and bitter about their medical experiences. Anecdotal observations made by clinicians may offer questionable snapshots of patients whose poor self-images, learning disabilities, and understandable anxiety often cause them to appear passive in "captive" medical situations.

From a research sample of fifty-six affected adults and twenty-five parents of affected children in Manchester, England, Benjamin et al. (1993) reported that NF1 had a "marked affect" on the lives of subjects and their families. Sixty-three percent of affected adults had experienced difficulties in school and 77 percent of parents reported such difficulties for their affected children. Forty-eight percent of the affected adults said that particularly the cosmetic aspects of the condition caused them anxiety during their adolescent years. Twenty-seven percent felt that learning difficulties experienced at school had caused problems with career attainment. Thirty percent felt that forming new contacts and relationships would be easier without their NF1. The majority of patients judged the severity of their conditions to be more serious than clinicians had judged them. The authors suggest that the impact of cosmetic features may be of more relevance to the individual than the clinical features that form the basis of clinicians' classifications.

FAMILY REACTION

NF1 may impact significantly on family life, and the greater the severity or visibility of symptoms, the more serious may be the impact. Any specific health condition of one family member may affect the total family emotional climate, behavior, and role expectations. However, a genetically transmitted disorder may have special meanings and may crucially affect family functioning in myriad ways.

Weiss and Mackta (1996), writing from many years of experience with individuals and families with diverse genetic conditions, describe common initial family responses:

Common to all is the initial shock that presages upheaval and irreversible change. Whether there is a definitive diagnosis or the unsettling knowledge that "something is wrong," it is necessary to go through an actual grieving process (Kubler-Ross, 1969). Grieving for the loss of a dream that includes having a perfect child, good health, or living happily ever after, everyone needs to go through stages, which can occur in any order: shock and denial, anger and resentment, bargaining and guilt, sadness and depression, and, finally, acceptance and coping with reality. Individuals move back and forth within these stages. (Weiss and Mackta 1996:24)

The public knows relatively little about genetics and the genetic transmission of conditions or diseases, and less about the various factors that can affect them. The names of most genetic disorders are difficult to pronounce, hard to remember, and even harder to spell. Consequently, families of an individual with a genetic disorder can be subject to additional stresses resulting from their own lack of understanding. The parents of an affected child may feel defective. They can be plagued by agonizing questions such as, What did I do wrong? Am I being punished for something I did or did not do? Affected individuals ask many of the same questions and can harbor troubling and distorted images of themselves and family members. (Weiss and Mackta 1996:26)

Three chapters in *Neurofibromatosis: A Handbook for Patients, Families, and Health-Care Professionals* (Rubenstein and Korf 1990) deal with psychosocial issues. Wilson and Yahr (1990) present an overview of issues and problems that families affected by NF1 might face. They note that the experience around the initial diagnosis might set the tone for the impact of NF1 on the family. They suggest that the timing of the diagnosis may be very important, with a diagnosis early in life auguring the best adjustment. The authors discuss the possible effect of the family on the individual with NF1 and conversely the effect of a member or members with the condition on the family, on family decision-making, and finances. The authors state that uncertainty may be the most difficult aspect of NF1 for families to cope with.

Wellman (1990) presents a general discussion of the impact of NF within the context of the varied problems, concerns, and needs of all adolescents in this society noting that, "NF complicates the period of adolescence—for those with very mild manifestations as well as for those with more serious problems" (Wellman 1990:211). Wellman focuses on issues of physical appearance, medical care, and adaptation. Likewise, Ellis (1990) discusses psychosocial aspects of appearance within the contexts of the general development of body image, social adaptation, and the importance of physical beauty and robust health and appearance in American society.

In one of the few articles attending to psychosocial issues of children with NF1 Counterman et al. (1995) reported on a study that examined perceived NF1 symptom severity and social support systems as correlates of psychological adjustment in seventeen children (fourteen African American and ten white). Children with more severe symptoms had a lower sense of self-worth and were dissatisfied with their behavior; yet, by parents' reports, the children with severe NF1 had fewer behavior problems. While children and parents agreed in their ratings of severity, they differed in their perceptions of the children's adjustments. The findings emphasize the importance of parents' and teachers' support for children's perceptions of themselves. The authors suggest that despite the evidence that support from parents and teachers can protect the children from negative psychological effects, parents may not be willing or able to see their child's distress.

Dilts et al. (1996) report that children with NF1 tended to be less competent than their siblings in a number of areas. The authors present a "behavioral phenotype" for NF1, referring to relationships among the biological and social characteristics in a given syndrome. The authors state:

Family dynamics probably contribute to the NF1 profile. Physical and psychological differences between children with NF1 and unaffected siblings become a part of the family's social context. Parents may tend to evaluate their children in relation to other children in the immediate or extended family as opposed to children in general. In this context, the parent may perceive the child with NF1 as low functioning.

Parents' expectations and attitudes may be internalized by the child and either interfere or facilitate the child's development. . . .

It is the complex of multiple factors that distinguishes the behavioral phenotype of NF1. We propose that the child's competencies, appearance, and physical disease factors interact with the social context, and these interactions contribute to the "psychosocial burden" of NF1 (Riccardi 1992). The diverse and interactive nature of problems encountered by children with NF1 suggests that active prevention interventions and anticipatory guidance will be needed to minimize the psychological consequences of NF1 to the child and other family members. (Dilts et al. 1996:238)

Ventmiglia and Balestrazzi (1996) report clinical findings and issues of daily life of families with NF1 who spanned many regions of Italy. Among topics covered are issues of health, management, social life, procreative decision-making, problematic barriers of daily life, and support systems. While some of the parents were also affected, the focus of this research is on affected children.

My own publications (Ablon 1992a, 1995, 1996, 1998) have outlined a host of problems and anxieties experienced by many affected adults and parents of affected children. Within the context of unpredictability of the disorder and rigid societal prescriptions for beauty, many subjects struggled with fears of disfigurement as well as medical problems. The issues faced by adults will be presented more fully in this volume.

This review of the literature on psychosocial issues suggests that a broad range of problems may be experienced by persons with NF1, such as those caused by physical symptoms that may compromise personal appearance, or issues around learning disorders and associated cognitive competencies. Societal stigma that may be a source and consequence of these problems has a serious impact on self-image, self-esteem, and social relationships. However, it should be kept in mind that there is a gamut of responses to NF1, and the literature reviewed above focuses on problems experienced. Persons who have few problems with their condition may not come to the attention of clinicians or researchers. As is true with other genetic conditions, psychosocial issues have received very little research or interventionist attention in comparison with clinical concerns. The following chapters provide a window on the experiences of daily life confronted by persons with this complex genetic disorder.

3

Diagnosis and Family Response

Most of the fifty-four affected adults could report on the approximate time and circumstances of the diagnosis of their NF1. A broad range of ages at diagnosis were reported:

Infancy–5	(early childhood)	8
6–12	(later childhood)	8
13–19	(teenage years)	18
20–29	(young adulthood)	8
30+	(adulthood)	12

There was little correlation between severity of subjects' condition (either in their youth or at present) and the time of diagnosis. It would appear that factors entering into very early diagnosis were visibility of symptoms, parents' willingness to take children for medical diagnosis and treatment, and access to and quality of medical care. Of those few whose diagnosis was made at birth or very early, one person's serious irregularity in one eye was apparent at birth. Others exhibited numerous cafe-au-lait spots. One said she had "pink spots" all over. In four instances subjects with an early diagnosis had mothers or fathers who were affected, but only one of these four was diagnosed at birth. The others were diagnosed at two years or older.

Eight persons were diagnosed from age six to twelve, all in divergent circumstances. Two had developed highly visible scoliosis, and others had likewise serious symptoms. Although five of these eight persons' mothers had the condition, this did not ensure an early diagnosis. Harry's mother, one of the few parents who talked openly about her NF1 condition to her affected son throughout his life, was likewise the only parent clearly reported to have diagnosed her son, even in the face of doctors' denials. Harry said:

I can remember that my mother came in to wash my back when I was in the tub one night and she saw the tumor on my hip. She was terrified. And we knew that was it. I guess she knew at birth because the doctor just kept on giving her excuses. I had one eye that was squinting down, and my left toe was deformed and she kept asking the doctor and he says, "No, no, no, no." I think she knew then.

They wouldn't even talk about it? What did they say about the cafe-au-lait spots?

It's "birthmarks."

Many other subjects talked about their multiple cafe-au-lait spots or tumors that appeared in childhood but these rarely led to the diagnosis of NF1. Maureen said:

I just remember when I was young, these freckles were on my torso, a lot of them there. My stepfather used to kid me about the spots. He told me they were "grasshopper spots." You know how when you pick up a grasshopper you will get the little brown spots? I guess everybody at that time just thought, "I guess she just has a lot of birthmarks."

Marilee talked about her childhood memories of her NF1: "My earliest recollection is when I was about seven. The kids would ask if I had been burned in a fire. It was then that I noticed what were cafe-au-lait marks on my back. I started asking my mom why the spots were there. She didn't know."

Doctors tended to display as much puzzlement about the cause of the cafe-au-lait spots and early tumors as did parents or peers. Said Jim:

The first doctor I saw said, "You have those brown spots. They have those spots in the more eastern states like Louisiana. Some people there commonly have them." He was from the South. He didn't know at the time what they were.

Eighteen persons were diagnosed in their teenage years. In several cases there was an accumulation of problems that culminated in diagnosis. Lily, who had many bumps on her scalp, remembers a series of doctors probing her. A physician in 1941 performed a biopsy on a fatty little tumor "like a jelly bean," however, "as long as we knew it wasn't cancer, nobody bothered with it." When Lily was eighteen she had a physical examination for entrance to college, and then at that time she first heard her condition named. The nurse asked if Lily had any cafe-au-lait marks after she mentioned having tumors, and Lily responded, "Yes, I have a big one right here on my pubic area, one on my breast, and on my arm." The nurse said, "The chocolate marks, 'cafe-au-lait,' come in conjunction with von Recklinghausen Disease." That was the first time she had ever heard this disease named. She was eighteen at the time.

Sarah commented bitterly on the failure of the medical profession to diagnose her despite her many symptoms:

I had all sorts of physical problems but I wasn't diagnosed till I was fourteen. My parents were frustrated, and they seemed to agree that there was something wrong. I suppose that they had a lot of faith in the medical personnel "who knew it all." *They* were educated, went to college, so they must know. And I was very frustrated at looking so strange and knowing that there was something wrong. There was no doubt in my mind that there was something wrong, but I was told continually that there was nothing wrong. I just knew that wasn't true. I never once believed that there was nothing wrong.

Hal, who worked in his yard a lot, was diagnosed at sixteen when his mother, who also had NF1 but was only diagnosed after Hal was, took him to the doctor because his back was bothering him.

My mother said, "Let's find out if you did something to yourself." The doctor said, "You just have a stiff back. I can't find anything physically wrong with you that caused you to be really sick, but has anyone ever told you that you have von Recklinghausen's Disease?" I said, "No." He said, "Well, you just have those few on your arms and the rest of your body and they don't seem to be bothering you, so don't worry about it."

Hal has since had several back surgeries to remove spinal tumors and a leg amputated because of a malignant tumor.

Four persons recounted dramatic physical events in the teenage years which they related to the first major manifestations of their condition. For example, in Robbie's case the diagnosis was made following an accident:

When I was thirteen I was in an automobile accident and I was in a body cast for a few months. When they took the body cast off, the lesions were on my chest and back. They weren't there before. Shortly after that I started having the parade of surgeries.

Benjamin recounted:

When I was fourteen years old I went swimming one day at a good friend's house and I got real, real weak, and as I was walking upstairs to my room I got violently sick and coughed up all this blood. And within two days I was in emergency surgery and they removed a neurofibroma, a bleeding neurofibroma out of my chest cavity. I'd vomited so hard that I snapped the appendix too. They just found the appendix just sitting right on top of my ribs. The neurofibroma was about the size of a golf ball. Since then I've had them as large as soft balls and as small as a little pea removed out of me.

The other two persons recounted stories of their parents withholding details on even the existence of their condition. Said Michael, a spirited man, who talked about his active teenage years:

I didn't find out about the severity of it until about two years ago [at age thirty-three]. When I was in high school I used to race motorcycles. I had a real bad crash one time. About four, five months later after the crash, I started developing this severe pain in my left leg. I had to have surgery on my leg. I was under the impression that the surgery I had on my leg was related to the injuries from the motorcycle accident. I was kind of buffaloed into believing that I had had this hairline fracture on my leg and the surgery that they were doing was just to remove calcium deposits off my leg because my leg healed wrong because it had never been in a cast.

You said, "buffaloed." Were you told that?

I was told that by my mom. My mom and my doctor kind of got together. It wasn't the motorcycle accident. It was a neurofibromatosis growth on the bone of my leg. I had surgery twice. The first time I had surgery, I had a fifty-fifty chance of coming out of it losing my leg because of where the tumor was and the size of the tumor. It was the size of an orange. My mom just told me this two years ago when my son had to have surgery. My chin hit the floor. But then again, it's over; it's done with. The surgery worked. I've got both legs. I don't ride motorcycles anymore. I ride bicycles.

Terry spent much of our two long interview sessions recounting her parents' elaborately planned secrecy around her condition. When she was twelve she fell in gym class and wrenched her neck badly. Prior to that time she had experienced no pain.

I remember that it was a couple of months later that I started to get a lot of pain in my neck and I was really unable to turn it for long periods of time. I remember it hurt and I felt it and there was this really large tumor here. You can see this scar. The doctors I've talked to say that they have never heard of cases of trauma like that causing it. But the only thing I can recollect starting it was that fall I had in junior high.

Although Terry thinks she was diagnosed at birth, her parents refused to speak with her about the matter. Despite multiple surgeries, biopsies, biannual visits to doctors, and having her cafe-au-lait spots scrutinized by medical residents, "no one ever told me what was going on. I didn't know I had NF until I was almost twenty years old." Although Terry was in constant pain and "knew there was something wrong," no one would tell her why she hurt so. Her parents apparently instructed her doctors not to tell her what it was and they called it a "nervous condition."

I was told to believe that it was psychological. To a thirteen year old in pain, to be told that it was a "nervous condition," and I was a relatively intelligent thirteen year old, I thought it was psychological, totally. At that time, at the teenage years of my life, I was so unstable, so unbalanced that I had no idea what was going on and I had not the presence of mind to ask.

Why do you think of yourself as having been more unstable than any other thirteen year old?

Because I was in constant pain and I was constantly being told that I was wrong, that I didn't hurt, that it was all in my head. I was told to stop making something out of nothing, to stop making my parents miserable by complaining or telling them that I hurt. They said, "We don't believe you; stop telling us these things; we don't want to hear them." This was terrible for a teenager in junior high who can't turn her head, and I literally couldn't. It was from one very large tumor that was pressing up against some kind of muscle. It was extreme pain.

When Terry was twenty and in college she went to see a doctor, to ask about some of her symptoms.

He said, "That's because of your NF." I said, "My what?"

How did he explain it?

I was in such a state of shock for a long time that I actually blanked it out. He talked about it being a genetic disease. He gave me a couple of prognoses like, "You'll be deaf by the time you're thirty and blind by the time you're forty." Very, very definite stuff like that.

Two men who were diagnosed at age eighteen described contrasting responses to their condition. Luis candidly talked about his depression and withdrawal in response to his diagnosis at age eighteen. "I guess I wasn't able to understand much at that time, or I didn't bother to. I didn't want to have anything to do with it, but I couldn't get it out of my mind. It was just frustrating. I guess that's what got me into drugs."

In contrast, Todd reported a much more casual response to the diagnosis and information he received when he was eighteen. Although he had numerous cafe-au-lait spots and skin tumors as a child, he had not been diagnosed previously.

The doctor mentioned that I didn't have a whole lot to worry about, but that it would cause a few troubles now and then. I didn't really think about it a whole lot until I started getting more and more bumps all the time. And when we had the last of our three children we noticed that he had cafe-au-lait spots. Then I started thinking about it a lot.

Three persons stated that doctors had made very general or fuzzy comments about their conditions, but these apparently did not register as a giving them a named condition or the idea that they should have any potentially serious concern. These persons only vaguely remembered the occasions.

Eight persons who were diagnosed between the ages of twenty and twenty-nine represent some of the mildest cases as well as several of the most extreme in terms of severity and visibility. The following accounts of diagnosis were presented by Rhoda and Florence, two very mildly affected women, both of whom have very severely affected adult children. Neither perceived their doctors' statements as predictive of serious problems for their offspring. Said Rhoda:

I was about twenty-four or twenty-five. I was working for a large company and went to their doctor because of these few little bumps. He removed one and told me it was von Recklinghausen.

What did the doctor tell you about the condition?

He said, "Maybe you shouldn't have children because the children will have it," but I don't remember him telling me what the consequences were that they could be anything more than the lumps I had. And if the lumps didn't bother me, why should they bother anybody? I hardly knew I had them. So I didn't think anything more about it.

Florence was married and had two children when she found out about her condition. Prompted by her father's having had cancer, she visited a free cancer clinic.

This doctor had me stark naked out on the examining table, and I have all these little bumps all over, and he says, "My, you are the best case of von Recklinghausen Disease I have seen in a long time." Of course I was scared. What do I have? He says, "Oh, it's just like all these little tumors you have on you, these little tiny little things; you really don't have anything to worry about. Oh, not to worry." So I never thought anything more about it.

The doctor did not tell her that she had a genetic disorder, and Florence did not connect her condition with her mother's having multiple cafe-au-lait spots.

Two other women were in their twenties and pregnant at the time of diagnosis. One woman was in her fifth month of pregnancy. The doctor angered her by telling her that she had NF and should not be pregnant. Another woman tells of receiving her diagnosis:

We went to the gynecologist to find out how far along I was and he referred me to a genetic counselor. We just walked in and he said, "Okay, you have this von Recklinghausen Disease and you have a fifty-fifty chance of having a normal child and a fifty-fifty chance you'll have one with problems. You could have optic nerve tumors; you could have brain tumors; you could have mental retardation; you could have tumors in the ears and thus hearing problems. Any of the problems that I am talking about that your child could encounter are the same problems that you could encounter." Then he advised me to have an abortion.

Here you go in and you are very excited about being pregnant and then you are told that these are the problems that you could encounter and there is no guarantee at all. It is like taking the dice and shaking it and not knowing if your child is going to come out with or without these problems and if it doesn't have them early, it could mature into these problems. My husband and I decided that this was not what we wanted so we had the pregnancy terminated.

How far along were you?

Three months. Or, actually, it was two months and you spent the next month crying.

Twelve persons were diagnosed in their thirties or later, two of these in their fifties. In this group of twelve are some of the more severely affected and visible as well as the most lightly affected. One woman was diagnosed during childbirth and three others only at the time that their children were diagnosed. Recounted Jody whose baby came early when she was away on vacation:

They did a caesarian. Later I was told that I had a growth on my hip and they had also removed that during surgery. They just wanted to see what it was. The next day came four or five doctors, all in white coats with their clipboards. One of them told me that they had tested the growth and they had found neurofibromatosis. I didn't understand what that was. They finally said it was The Elephant Man's Disease and told me it was hereditary. They had checked and the baby had it. She had a number of large cafe-au-lait marks on her trunk. There I was in the situation of finding out I had this strange disease and my child did too. Everything was very shocking with the baby being taken a month and a half early and then finding all this out!

Laura described the sequence of events that followed the diagnosis of her five-year-old son who had had many medical problems:

Dr. McGee started counting all the cafe-au-lait spots and marking them with a pen and then he asked me if I had them and how many do I have. And I told him, "A lot," and he said, "How large are they?" and I said, "Some are quite large" and that's when he told me that he thought it was von Recklinghausen Disorder and that it was the same thing as The Elephant Man's Disorder. The doctor advised me 100 percent against having more kids. He said that I had a fifty-fifty chance of having another child with NF. And he said, "I advise you to go straight to your gynecologist and have your tubes tied."

And Isabelle, who was a quadriplegic at the time of interviewing, had gone to a doctor many years before when she was having trouble walking.

I was lurching, so I went to the doctor. He told me I had The Elephant Man's Disease. I knew about The Elephant Man and I figured that I was going to get these big lumps on me and be grotesque and that I would be a freak. He about as much told me that. He said I had a lot of tumors, thousands of tumors inside. I do have some on my face and on my arms, you know, all over, but they're not as noticeable as some people's. I've never met anybody else personally with NF, I've just seen it on TV. But when I talked to Dr. Simmons and he told me I had The Elephant Man's Disease I figured that's what was going to become of me, and I was suicidal at the time because I didn't want to do that to my husband or my family. I didn't want to be grotesque. I'm not a beautiful woman, but I'm an attractive woman.
Dr. Simmons believed in being very straight and not hiding anything or beating around the bush. And he sat me down and said, "Well, this is going to happen, and that's going to happen, and you'll get these grotesque lumps and pretty soon you'll be in a wheelchair for the rest of your life." He was right about part of it, but not until about fifteen years later. I had fifteen years where I didn't have to be in a wheelchair.
So how did you feel after he told you?
Oh, I wanted to die! I wanted to die! I didn't even want to tell my husband about The Elephant Man thing.

Two men were diagnosed in their fifties with serious tumors of the spine and brain. One had an immediate spinal surgery and was told he barely escaped paralysis. The second died from complications around his condition within the interview period, less than a year after his diagnosis.

EARLY FAMILY RESPONSE

"My father had a flawed baby," said Terry bitterly. "They knew when I was born that I had the disease. It was the dirty secret of the family. It was a *whispering disease*. I was never told. I don't even think my sister knew." Although her parents would speak to others about her condition, they still will not speak to Terry about it. When she tries to bring it up they tell her she is trying to ruin their lives and cause them heartache.

A significant literature documents the negative shock and varied sequelae resulting from the birth of a physically or mentally different child (Fortier and Wanlass 1984; Ablon 1988; Weiss and Mackta 1996). The earlier the diagnosis, the more dramatic may be family reactions. In the cases of the affected adults reported on here, the diagnoses spanned many years, and in fact only a small number of first generation subjects could report on the early responses of their parents to their NF1.

Some who had been diagnosed in infancy or early childhood recounted stories of parental guilt, shame, or mutual blame of each other for their child's condition. The concept that NF1 could be caused by a mutation was either not explained to parents, not well understood by them, or sometimes not known to physicians in past years. Parents often blamed themselves or each other for their child's condition. Even though affected persons today have been told that their NF1 could be the result of a mutation, they also sometimes still speak of "the one who gave it to me."

Lou, who had early serious spinal surgeries, described her parents as "really going through hell and blaming it on each other. I don't know if it's their egos or whatever, but I don't think they want to pinpoint who's the culprit for me getting it. It seems really strange. I just think they're both scared to find out who was the one that actually gave me this." When I reminded her that it may not be either one of them, she said, "Yeah, I know."

Several persons stated that one parent continually blamed themselves for the condition, but they were never tested to provide a basis for this belief.

Reggie, whose mother and father were in their early forties at the time of his birth, said that his father blamed himself for Reggie having NF1 because of the numerous x-rays that he had had as part of his having had tuberculosis. "There was always a high level of guilt on his part."

Most of those whose diagnoses were in the teenage or young adult years reported their parents did not worry significantly at the time. For example, said Theresa, "Once they were told it wasn't going to be cancer or anything like that, then as I remember, there wasn't a worry about it." And Elise:

They didn't react much to my NF. I think that was because my mother had so many of her own health problems. Hers were so real and there were problems right then.

I think that Mother and Dad's attitude was, "Elise has this—however you pronounce it—Recklinghausen, but she is fine. She's not having a problem so we don't need to discuss it with her." Probably, at that time I saw that as a lack of interest. It would have made me feel more important and more loved had they said, "Hey, let's see what's going on here, what we can do about this," which nobody did.

Subjects were asked if they received differential treatment because of their NF1. Most subjects stated that their parents did not treat them differently from their siblings. However they reported a wide range of early behaviors of their siblings toward them. For example, Darla, the closest sibling to Rosa, was four when Rosa's tibia first broke at ten months. The fracture occurred when Darla set Rosa down after picking her up.

I think she carried around a lot of guilt feelings in the beginning, saying she had broken my leg. But the tumor was already there, breaking, just deteriorating the bone. All of my brothers and sisters were really great when I was growing up. When I was little at the park, I would have on the cast or my brace and if some of the other kids were being mean to me my brothers and sisters would stick up for me. I can remember my brother saying, "I'm going to beat you up if you do anything."

In contrast is Sarah's memory: "My siblings never helped me. They tried to deny that the NF had any effect, and that if I had a pretty face I'd be complaining about something else. And it was always kind of discounted and denied."

These early behaviors often set the pattern for the quality of the relationships of adulthood.

CURRENT RELATIONSHIPS WITH FAMILY

Subjects reported a wide gamut of current relationships with their families. Many subjects' parents served as confidants, friends, and nurses at crisis periods. Three unmarried male subjects, among the most seriously affected in the sample, talked about the unswerving practical and emotional support of their parents. Said Benjamin, "If I was in terrible pain or despondent I would call my father or mother. We've really grown close over the last few years. My mom and I are best friends. And my dad's my second best friend. They have seen me go through a lot."

Said Randy:

My parents are real supportive. You can't really take care of yourself the first three or four weeks after you've had heavy surgery so my parents always have a place for me to stay, and there's always somewhere I can crash. The last time I stayed at my parents' for three weeks. I'm independent enough that as soon as I'm able to get up and drive, then I'm back at my own place.

And Nathan recounted, "When I was having difficult chemotherapies, my mother would come up after the chemotherapy treatments and stay with me for a week."

Accounts of current relationships with siblings reflected a broader range of attitudes and behavior, from those persons who reported a lifetime of great closeness and frequent interactions, to distance, indifference, and even hostility. For example, said Carrie, "My brother is the closest person in my life. When I was growing up, my brother was everything my father wasn't. My brother was there for me when I needed a brother. He was my friend when I needed a friend. He was everything. He still is." And Clarise, who both worked and socialized with her family:

My two sisters and I have talked about the fact that they would take care of me if anything ever happened to me. We're there for each other 100 percent all the time. It's really rare. Some people think we're very strange. [Laughing] And I don't know how it happened, how it evolved that way, but it just did.

However, more than half of the affected adults report a life of distance from their sibling or siblings. Citing reasons of differences in life style, or siblings' selfishness, laziness, or unlawful behavior, most of these stated they rarely or never see them. Several described distant older siblings who persecuted or "picked on" them or at best avoided them when they were children and still treat them condescendingly as adults. Said Chuck:

The only time my sisters were ever really attentive to me was when I was sick. Other than that it was just like, "We're doing something. You go over there and do something else." Even now though I make much less money than they do, they expect me to pay proportionately more than my share for gifts for our folks.

Said Jim:

When I was in the fifth grade in school my brother started to say, "Get lost. I don't want you around." He would do his homework in the bedroom and close the door. He wouldn't let me study in there. I had to study in the kitchen with the TV blaring in the living room. I had all these learning problems and then I got distracted by the TV all the time. Then I was living with my mother when she died. He wanted his half of the house right then if I wanted to stay there. I went to about ten loan companies trying to get money, but I'd have had payments of $550 a month to pay him off. That would have left me $50 a month to live on from my crummy job. Now he owns his own business in San Francisco. He still says, "Oh, get lost." That's how nasty he is.

Five women with serious and visible problems with their NF1 described siblings who did not support them in their times of need as children. These siblings, now as adults with no health problems, still can find no identity with the problems of the affected subjects. In some cases consciousness of the beauty and/or comfortable lifestyles of these nonaffected siblings contributes to subjects' own sense of failure or despondency about their fate in life. Their descriptions are vivid and telling. I asked Terry to describe her sister:

Beautiful, intelligent, witty. I mean, she's wonderful, she's a great person.

Are you close to her?

We are starting to get close. It was really hard for her growing up because I was the different one and I was always made to feel defective and she had to be extra perfect to cover for that. Since I was the defective one I was always set up to fail. But she had to be perfect.

She had no choice. She was made to be Daddy's perfect daughter because I was Daddy's defective daughter. It has been a lot of years but we are finally starting to get a kind of sisterly relationship.

And Lou:

My sister, she's so, how can I put it? The way she presents herself is appealing, attractive. She dresses well, she has nice posture and she gets stared at a lot by guys. She said she knows that sometimes she tries to block it out because it makes her feel uncomfortable. How could *that* make you feel uncomfortable, or make you feel weird? To me, I think that should make you feel good. How would you like to be just the opposite? Someone making fun of you or looking at you because you have a disfigurement like me.

A few weeks ago we went to the grocery store. And there's this guy kept staring at her. Once she even met a guy when they were both driving down the freeway. They pulled over and talked and she went out with him the next day. She could meet somebody just walking to work. She doesn't have no problem meeting men whatsoever.

That's why I don't like to go out with her. There's so many guys looking at her that it tees me off sometimes. Also she never knows what she wants to do. I said, "You are one of those people that are never satisfied." To me a person that can never be satisfied can never be happy in their life. If she had to go through what I went through she could never do it. I think she'd commit hari kari.

And Isabelle, who is a quadriplegic, describes a sister who can find no identity with her condition.

My sister is a social butterfly. Because nothing bad has ever happened to her, she's the kind of person who doesn't like to hear bad things. She very seldom comes here. Sometimes I start to cry and she just turns and says, "Oh, Isabelle, things aren't so bad. You have a nice home and you have someone that's taking care of you and things could be worse, you know." So I gave up trying to talk to her.

Seven affected adults reported one or more siblings with NF1. In three of these cases the interviews reflected a sympathy or closeness with these persons that may have been fostered by their common NF1 experiences. In two additional cases subjects speculated, based on the presence of learning disabilities and/or a marginal number of cafe-au-lait spots, that a sibling may have NF1 but denies it.

Fifteen of the affected adults in my sample, almost one-third, have very attenuated friendship or social support systems. In almost every case individuals who are not married rely on their parents for monetary and other significant practical support. Some of these are single adults in their thirties and forties who continue to live with their parents even when employed, or if they live separately, still rely on parents for economic support when they are unemployed or temporarily laid off. In most cases of the total fifteen and even of those few in this number who are married, relations with parents and siblings also appear to be their chief social contacts. In the two cases where the affected adult has broken off with parents or parents have refused support, one, Norita, has been accepted as a surrogate member by a family that has served as her advocate in employment disputes and assisted her at times of surgery. In the second case, Sarah, after leaving her second abusive husband, is now homeless. The small circle of friends maintained by these fifteen subjects appears to be due chiefly to their poor self-image and self-consciousness about their visible condition or learning disabilities, and to their lack of social skills. Five of the men speak of themselves as "loners" from childhood. These findings also underline the dependency of these affected adults, chiefly in the economic area, and point up the importance of and necessity for strong family support through the life course.

4

Intergenerational Sharing

Cecilia, a well-educated and lively woman in her thirties, spoke at length with me about the emotional dynamics surrounding the NF1 in her family:

I know it's not very nice but I've resented and hated my mother for a lot of years for giving NF to me. I looked at my mother, and I couldn't help but see this ugly woman, this disfigured ugly woman, and I wished she didn't have it because everybody else's mother was normal looking. When people said, "This is my mom," I used to feel a little bit of embarrassment to say, "This is *my* mom," because I didn't want anyone making any comments or asking any questions.

I have learned that it's not her fault. I can't really blame her; it's not like on purpose she said, "I want to give this to my daughter." I've been told that I will not necessarily have it as severely as my mother has. I used to think that would happen and it used to bum me out. I used to be convinced that I was going to be exactly like her. I mean we look alike—the same height, basically the same weight. Everything is the same about us. The same fat fingers. I've always thought, "Oh no, if I have everything else like my mother, I must really have her genes and I'm going to be as severely affected." But now I know that that's not true.

One significant component of the dysfunction that may occur when a family is challenged by genetic disorder is disruption or virtual absence of communication about the condition between parents and children. Relations between an affected parent and affected child or children may be severely damaged or compromised by the consequences of guilt, denial, or massive anger. In fact, researchers studying a variety of genetic conditions have documented the positive aspects of communication for education and emotional support, leading to enhancement of well-being and a diminished level of fears about the future (for example, Miller et al. 1986–1987).

Of the fifty-four affected adults in the sample, fifteen had a parent with NF1. In all but two cases this was a mother. Because the condition occurs equally in men and women, it is not clear why so few of the sample had affected fathers. However the fact that the great majority of subjects had inherited NF1 from their mothers may possibly have tilted the sample in the direction of severity. Articles by Miller and Hall (1978) and Hall (1990a) suggest that inheritance of NF1 from the mother might be associated with increased severity in keeping with the concept of "genetic imprinting," that is, "modifications of genetic material take place depending upon whether genetic information is derived from the mother or father" (Hall 1990a:2). While varied types of observations strongly suggest that in general this process might occur, no systematic evidence for this occurring in NF1 has demonstrated this clearly. In the two cases in the sample where the subject had inherited their condition from the father, both persons had conditions of mild severity, and in one case was moderately visibly affected and in the other mildly visibly affected.

Twenty affected adults, fifteen women and five men, have at least one affected child. Of these, six have two or more affected children. One person has four affected adult children. Four three-generational families are represented in this sample. Thus, a variety of points of view of the sharing of NF1 between generations was presented: second-generation adults' views of themselves as children and their affected parents, and adults' views of themselves and their affected children. A wide range of attitudes were expressed. These are highlighted below.

ADULT CHILDREN AND THEIR PARENTS

Most subjects who had affected parents had little specific knowledge about their parents' condition. There were many ambiguities surrounding their diagnosis. For example, Carrie's mother had gone to different hospitals trying to figure out what the growths were but nobody could give her an answer, nor did Carrie's mother know that Carrie had the same condition. Carrie was seventeen when her mother died. Carrie recounted:

They had no idea what it was. I later found out that my mother had it and that's how I got it. She had it bad. She had real big tumors on a lot of her body. Some were inside too.

But she never knew that she had NF in her life? What did she think she had?

She thought they were growths of some kind, but there wasn't a name to put to it. Nobody told her anything. Mine wasn't bad; I wasn't being too bothered by it. By the time I found out what I had, my mother had already died.

Michael told me about his mother's secrecy around her condition:

You see, mom doesn't really like to talk about it that much. That sometimes creates a problem because you can't break down the walls. You've got to work around it, go over the top to talk to her about it. But I am assuming that my mom was aware of it prior to my birth. This idea of passing it on from her to me is this thing that is kind of clouded. It is like, "I've got it and my mom has it and that's it; we don't talk about it."

When Nadine's son was born, she did not know about her own NF1. She thought his cafe-au-lait spots were birthmarks like her family had assumed her father's and her own spots were. And Florence:

I had a lot of little bumps and a few cafe-au-lait spots but no one wondered about them. My mother had several ones, and then she had several very peculiar tumor-like things on her side, and no one ever really diagnosed that as NF. In retrospect I'm quite sure her sister had it too, but it was never diagnosed.

Most adult subjects stated they did not blame their parents for passing on the condition, and were matter of fact about the situation—it was just something that happened from parent to child, the same as the likelihood of passing on hair color or body build. Most accepted the fact that their parents typically had scanty information about the condition. Chuck said:

I don't think I want to have blood children because I know what I could do to my children. But when Mom was having kids, they didn't know it was hereditary. She didn't have no idea what was going on. So I never really blamed her for what happens to me. But there is a higher power named God. I blame Him more than I blame anyone else. I blame Him more about my lot in life and I tell people I'm Murphy's Law incarnate. If it's going to happen, it's going to happen to me.

And Randy commented, "My mom blames herself a lot more than I blame her for what has happened to me."

Only one person, Cecilia, expressed current serious resentments toward her mother. It is possible that others harbored similar resentments earlier in their lives or even currently, but were not inhibited in expressing them to me than was Cecilia. Cecilia's account reflects some of the many issues of contemporary life and society that have interacted with their or their parents' concerns around NF1.

As you were growing up did you think of how NF affected your mother's life?

Not when I was younger. Not when I was between sixteen and twenty-one. I have to admit I was selfish, and only thought of how it affected me. I resented her for giving it to me. But I couldn't help it. When I did go to therapy over these past nine years, I've talked about it a lot. All I thought of was me—how it affected me. I wasn't bright enough or sensitive enough to think of how it affected her.

Would she talk about it very often?

No. But, when I was in the dating age, she used to say things like, "Look, your father loves me. When a man loves you, they love you for what's inside." So she never really talked about it. Once I was covering up a scar and she says to me, "Why would you do that?" I mean, I think it's pretty obvious why you would want to cover up a scar with make-up. So she would say things that led me to believe that it didn't bother her.

I have to admit that sometimes I feel bad that, gee, I never really thought about how it affected her. And she must feel bad for giving it to me. Because everybody wants to have a normal, healthy, perfect child. And I didn't really think of those things. But then I don't get too hard on myself, because I can't change the past. I didn't consider her, I only thought of me, and that's what I needed to do to survive, I think. I got angry, I resented.

I've talked about it with my sister and some of the boyfriends that I've had. It's helped me that some of the therapists that I've gone to and some of the articles that I've read say that it's very normal for me to resent my mother. She did give it to me. So, I'm not proud that I've hated my mother, but it's something I'm going to have to cope through. And I have.

Do you think it has made it harder or easier for you that your mom has it?

Harder. Of course I don't know that for sure, because I didn't have a mother that didn't have it.

Why do you think it's harder?

With mutation, they might have doted over me, tried to take me to the doctors. But it was harder for me because by the time I was thirteen, my mom already had it. As I was getting older, I was getting more aware. I was getting interested in boys and I saw that my mother had it. Not talked about, and then I started to come with it. And obviously I knew where I got it from; I got it from my mother.

This isn't very nice. But I already started to look at my mother and be repulsed, because it is ugly. It wasn't nice of me, but I went by looks. And I had a hard time looking at her and then thinking to myself, "Oh my God, I hope I don't look like that. I'd kill myself." And then sure enough, I did start to get it.

Other things started to play into my mom's and my relationship. Like everybody else in the seventies, I started drinking beer, smoking marijuana, and all the kind of stuff that drove her crazy. She thought I was going to turn into a tramp. So she had those resentments against me. She couldn't just let me be. She didn't trust me. And here I had this against her, because I had a hard time looking at her, and I resented her because she was giving me NF. We never talked about it. So that didn't help. And I never had my mother go, "Oh, it's okay, you get used to it." Or, "It's not that bad, you know." I never heard her say any of those things to make me feel that it was okay, and that I was still going to live.

It appears that many of those who have had parents with NF1 have not had helpful role models for living with NF1. Many second-generation NF1 subjects report a total lack of communication about NF1 with their parents. Essentially, they have encountered a stone wall. "I never had one discussion with my mother about it," said Annie.

My mother never talked about it. And she made it clear she didn't want to talk about it.

When you were growing up did you ask her what she had?

No. I think we were like kind of afraid to. We never talked about it. It was always just like kind of hidden and when I would talk about it, I was just kind of told "God had a reason for this." "God," you know, like "God was the one responsible."

And Michael: "I tried to talk to my mom about it and sure, she would give me a couple of answers, like, 'Here, that will shut him up.' Then she goes on to another subject."

Two persons spoke of the severity of their mothers' conditions and described how their observation of these strong women coping heroically with significant physical handicaps assisted them into becoming fighters for themselves and their children. Harry, a severely and visibly affected man, often talked about his mother. They had spoken freely about their shared NF1.

I guess I can thank my mother for my attitudes. My mother had a lot of pain with her NF. She walked on two crutches all over the country before she went into a wheelchair. I was raised the same way. You see, if you can't do it one way, you can do it another way. My mom helped me to know handicapped people. I've been around handicapped people all my life. There's an old saying I grew up with, I guess. I lived by it, pretty well. "I felt sorry I had no shoes 'till I saw a man who had no feet." I think, "Gee, how would I feel if I were in that person's shoes?" There's always somebody worse. Just deal with people the way they are, accept it for what they are, not for what they look like or because they are missing a few things.

Besides having NF1, Leah's mother had lost a leg due to another health problem. Nonetheless, she raised three children and inspired Leah to view her as challenged, not handicapped.

You know, I would look at my mom and see a very normal person. I never saw her handicap. When people would tell me that my mom was handicapped, I would answer, "No she's not." To this day I don't like that word. I hate to hear, "Poor thing, she's handicapped." I would prefer to say that she was "challenged." She was not handicapped. She was able to have three children and raise them and all three of us turned out perfectly well, outside of a little minor NF.

Others spoke of pitying their mothers' highly visible conditions and feared their own NF1 might someday become as serious a problem. Grace found her fear increasing as she aged and rarely visited her parents because she was scared. "I don't want to be reminded of what my mother is going through right now. And yet I know I should, because she brought me up. She could use some kind of support herself."

Peter spoke to me often about his very visibly affected mother:

I found out that NF affects the person as far as their thinking is concerned. My mom don't think that clear. She's smart and she's strong. It's not like she's retarded or nothing. It's just like she doesn't know how to dress herself. She never did know how to talk; she was a loner. For years I was ashamed to recognize that was my mother. Now I say, "So what? If you don't like it, take a walk." She's just been from heck. There hasn't been a day of her life that she hasn't had to do some paying for the NF. I hope mine never gets that bad.

Subjects did not feel that their affected parent raised them differently than their siblings despite their sharing of NF1. Randy commented:

I don't think my mom raised me differently because of the NF. I think I was raised differently because I was the baby of the family. Also I think it was more because of the hyperactivity that they treated me differently.

Harry, on the other hand, did think his mother raised him differently from his brother:

My mom raised me having more independence and doing more. My brother had a lot done for him. I was allowed to be more independent, to do things on my own. She trained me that way. I guess she thought I needed to learn to handle more. Since I couldn't rely on anyone else I would have to rely on myself.

Sometimes you hear that if a child has a particular health condition the parents might be protective toward that child, but you are saying that this was the opposite.

Yeah, the opposite, and I am meeting people in special education at the college who are being treated the same way. Their parents are saying, "Ah, hah! You are this way, and it's too bad, but you are going to have to learn to do it yourself." It is great. It is more difficult than being raised normal.

AFFECTED ADULTS AND THEIR CHILDREN

A range of attitudes was expressed by affected adults about their responsibility in passing on their condition to their children. Attitudes varied from matter-of-fact-ness to guilt. Many parents expressed guilt. "Oh, I have guilt. If I had it to do over again I would not have children. You know, they all have it," said Regina. This mother's responsibility for passing on NF1 to them was frequently brought up by her children. "One of my daughters said that she did not want any of her school friends to know about the NF. Her sister said, 'Why not? Why are you ashamed of it? It's not your fault.' I said to them, 'No, it's not your fault.' And Lee said, 'No. It's not our fault, it's *your* fault!' "

Grace also spoke about the emotional problems around the condition in their three-generational NF1 family:

You know, I've been thinking about this lately, since my children are having to deal with it and I have not really dealt with it in my life enough that I think that I'm on top of it. I know my children are very angry. Well, I guess I am, too, but maybe I'm a different type of person. When I ask my son about it, he says he's angry at grandma and I say, "You shouldn't be angry at grandma. If anybody, you should be angry at me." They won't discuss it with me. And they never would go to a [support group] meeting with me.

At least I'm admitting to myself that I'm angry about something, even if I haven't really found out or admitted what I'm angry about. I don't think I'm angry at my mother. I am angry at myself for bringing my children into the world with this condition. I feel bad about that, guilty. And sometimes I probably must feel, "Why me?" That's a real hard feeling. My children feel that.

Carl's very angry. He's hit me and even threatened to kill me. He said that his brother and he had made a pact, that if they got too bad they were going to kill themselves. Now, as to that, there's nothing I can do about it, if I can't get them to go to a counselor to try to become accepting and be able to live with it.

I am trying to push them into knowing more about it just so they have the knowledge. I've told them, "You have to get genetic counseling. You can't have children unless you really know what you're doing. It's a possibility." And at least they have that knowledge that I didn't really have or I should have had. Maybe if I had been a little bit more intelligent, had gone out and sought the knowledge, but, either way, it's done.

Six of the twenty affected adults who have affected children have one or more children who are significantly more seriously affected than they, with spinal, eye, and varied internal tumors. However the attitudes of these parents spanned the same range of attitudes as those parents with minimally affected children. Rhoda, who is only lightly affected, talked to me about passing NF1 on to two much more severely affected children. "When they told me, it was so early I wasn't dating at the time. And after seven years, it just slips your mind, or if I ever did know, I didn't think about it." Consequently she did not have information about NF1 to influence her when she became pregnant.

How did you feel about this when you really began to see that it could be something serious?

Well, I don't know. It's just like everything else. So you have to wear glasses. It's just one of those things. What are you going to do about it? I don't know whether I felt bad about it, that I had passed it on. But once it happened, there's nothing you can do about it, so why worry about it?

Do you think either of the kids has been resentful?

I've asked them, and they said, "No, why should I? I mean, some people have this and some people have that. After all, people pass everything on without knowing." Sometimes I think Hal is angry, and other times I'm not sure. I've asked him, "Do you blame me?" He says, "No, I don't blame you." What else can he tell his mother?

Corroborating her perspective, Hal confirmed that he did not blame his mother:

My mother keeps asking, "Do you blame me for having a kid, because you have this?" I say, "Mom, you didn't know, so just forget about it. And even if you did know, you only had that one bump, and how bad could one bump be?"

And another mother, when discussing the severity of her adult son's condition, stated:

I don't think I'll have any more problems. I mean, I'm getting old, and it's not going to kill me. But I worry for my son, Jacob. I don't know how much further this'll go in him, and I'm devastated by it. I still feel, not guilty, but I *can* feel guilty. It's not my fault; it's just one of those things. But I'm devastated for him and there's nothing I can do about it. For myself, I got a doctor that watches every little thing I do. But for Jacob, I worry about him. My husband talks to me and says I shouldn't allow myself to, it's not my problem; it's his. And he knows how to take care of it. It's his life and he knows how to handle himself; he knows what he has to do. And he has a good doctor.

Most of the affected parents queried about possible differences in their child-rearing practices stated that they did not think they were raising their affected children any differently than their other children or than they would had the children not had NF1. Said one mother, "I am not raising them any differently than I would have if they didn't have it or if I didn't have it. The only thing that I am going to focus on more than I would have normally because of their NF is the medical side of it." And another: "No. I don't think I am raising them differently. I may have to be more sensitive maybe to their fears because of it."

Nonetheless, other mothers thought they did treat their children differently. Said Sarah, who was often given to sensitive analyses of her situation:

I think sometimes it makes a lot of difference. And in terms of difficulty for both of us, it can make it easier sometimes and much harder at others.

How does it make it easier?

She knows she has somebody to relate to. It isn't somebody giving her lip service, and saying, "Yeah, I know how you feel." Somebody that does indeed, know. Somebody that has that experience. It's not so much that she may have the exact same feelings, although she may have, but she does get a sense of knowing that I know how she feels. And she knows that I understand when she comes home and somebody has been making fun of her for her spots.

Does she get angry about the NF or that you gave her NF?

No, she hasn't said that. She's just angry at having it. But she doesn't seem to be angry at me. It's just anger that she has it. She has lots of spots and scoliosis. She doesn't seem to be bothered as much as I was when I was a kid, but then, mine showed on my face, so unless I wore a paper bag, they could see it. I didn't wear paper bags. That could be that kind of difference. It could be bad for us if something would happen that it would make her feel physically deformed. Then I can see that it could cause problems for our relationship. She might be angry at me for causing her to have NF.

And another mother thoughtfully said:

Since I don't have the kind of problems that she has, I think just being knowledgeable about it is important. I try to be understanding of what she's dealing with. But I really haven't had the physical problems that she's had. If I had some more severe problems I don't know if I'd be more sympathetic with what she's dealing with. Hopefully what she has won't get a lot worse, but I foresee that if she's got this many problems now, from what little I've learned about NF, that she may be in for some hard times as she goes through puberty and as she gets a little bit older.

But, you know, I don't think we treat her that differently and we try to be empathetic when we need to be and boost her confidence, that even though she's got this cosmetic problem with her eye, that she's still a neat little girl and we love her and we try to make her feel good about herself.

Affected parents appeared to be very open about their condition and tried to educate their children about it, and also be sensitive to their emotional concerns. As Theresa told me:

I worked very hard in instilling in my children self-confidence and trying to tell them to feel good about themselves. Where I was aware of not really feeling good about myself because I didn't feel I looked as good as somebody else did. For that reason it's really important to me to try to instill confidence in all of them.

The attitudes of these affected parents greatly contrasted with those that second-generation adults reported for *their* parents in the subjects' growing up years. For example, in the home of Elise where NF1 was a frequent topic of conversation, when I visited, the children—all teenagers—would ask about the findings of my research. Elise told me: "We've always talked about the NF with them. We have made a point of giving them information all the way long. Even when they were little and they'd say, 'What are these spots that we have on our bodies?' we would tell them about it. Also, when my younger daughter was four or five, she had several surgeries and we told her exactly what was happening."

Luanne, another mother, expressed perhaps the most common sentiment of concern that affected parents feel for their affected children, "You want to know how NF affects people's lives? For me, it is not knowing what is going to happen to me or to my kids, particularly Rebecca. I often think, 'My God! Let it all happen to me, but let them be all right!' "

The situation of affected parents is a difficult one. They experience the unpredictability in two ways: from their own experiences and fears, and through their fears about the future health of their children. Further, affected parents do not necessarily exhibit more efficacy in managing their children's conditions. These parents, while more in tune with the kinds of problems their children might have or develop, frequently have suffered from learning disabilities. These have hindered their own education, resulting in low levels of school and occupational achievement and in poor self-image. In stressful situations such as medical encounters, these characteristics alone can produce the seemingly "gentle and docile" behavior that doctors have described for NF1 patients. Such parents are often not equipped for aggressive problem solving and asserting themselves in battles with doctors, school administrators and teachers, and hence, for the successful management of their children's conditions.

However, affected parents today are considerably more knowledgeable about their own condition and genetic disorders in general than were their parents' generation. This knowledge has released them from some of the guilt, fear, and religious attribution that may have enveloped their parents and led to secrecy and an unwillingness to discuss their shared condition. Most parents today are making every effort to be emotionally and practically available for their children and are attempting to educate them as much as possible about NF1.

5

The School Years—The Staging Ground for Stigma

Sarah often talked about her painful school experiences:

As a child when I was growing up and my self-esteem was forming, everything was being forced. At school, I would get shoved up against the wall by the boys and told I was "ugly" and "stupid" and "no good." They would say that I belonged in a freak show. Then I'd go home and again be told I was stupid. I started to think that I was stupid and ugly, not worth anything. So I went around with my head hung down. My grades were awful.

For all children the school years represent the first major interface with the social norms and public scrutiny of American society. These years are critical not only for preparing children educationally but for representing the chief arena for significant social development and interaction. The imprint of these years may vitally affect all the rest of a child's life in relation to knowledge and social skills and abilities.

Children who exhibit physical, cognitive, or lifestyle differences often find the school years a harrowing time. Pressures for achievement and conformity may bring forth problems with teachers and other students alike. A great many children with NF1 encounter serious problems throughout their school career. Slightly over one-half of the adults in my sample, twenty-eight out of fifty-four, report significant learning disorders during their school years. This proportion is consistent with studies reported in the literature (Rubenstein and Korf 1990, and many others). While today many children with NF1 are being monitored closely by their parents, and those with special needs are often in programs for the educationally handicapped, as mandated by Public Law 94-142, in the school years of my adult subjects—fifteen to fifty or more years ago—many were not diagnosed with NF1. Even in the cases of those who were diagnosed, it was not recognized that learning disorders commonly accompanied the condition. Those who reported disorders performed poorly in school and were typically labeled as "dumb" or "lazy." When I asked subjects how they remembered their school years, almost invariably they responded with negativity. They told remarkably similar tales of frustration and failure. Said Elise:

When I was five years old, my teacher told my mother I was a "moron." She wasn't saying it as a joke. She meant it. But just that night something happened in the kitchen and I saved my mother from seriously burning something. My mother knew that a "moron" could not have done that. I had to have intelligence to have done that. I did awful in school. I made poor grades and was told that I could not do certain things and that I maybe couldn't finish. When I graduated, they told me that I absolutely was not university material.

Michael, too, had painful memories of his school days:

I was always cast in remedial or one step above the remedial classes. And all of my friends were in the average or academic classes. It was always hard to have people think of me as a dummy. It was frustrating because I did not feel that I was dumb, like some of the kids in the dumb-dumb classes. They were airheads or punks or hoods. I knew I was above these guys, but with the information down in front of me, I couldn't compete. It was like I was trying to say, "Help me, do something." It was so embarrassing. I knew that I was better than these people were, but I couldn't change the way I performed. I have this memory of crying out for help, but maybe I wasn't crying out properly.

Once I had a paper put up on the board at school. It wasn't the best paper in the world but it was up there. My mom and dad were there for open house, and my dad looked at me and said, "Aw, gee, Mike, you can't even spell your own name right." You see, I've always had this problem with spelling. I had spelled my name wrong on the paper.

Subjects reported poor comprehension and spelling and reading skills. Despite the desire to learn, some individuals simply could not master reading. To this day several hate and avoid reading. Many say they could not pass a test because they could not remember anything. For example, said Claire:

My comprehension was low. I would read a page over and over again, to figure out what the page was talking about. I hated reading. I used to make a joke out of it. I used to equate it with taking out the garbage. Even today it is only something I will do if I have to.

Several subjects spoke with frustration about the problems around resources and the lack of special education programs available when they were in school. Said Michael:

The problem was in parochial school. I was in a class of medium size for the school, fifty-five students. The first year I had a lay teacher, he told my mother that since the class was so big, he couldn't give me individual instruction, that the advanced and the slow were going to suffer. He had to teach to the middle of the road and that if I couldn't keep up, then that's the way it was going to have to be.

Very few had parents able to pay for private assistance. Robbie talked about his experiences in elementary school:

My parents knew I had a learning disability. They did not press it in the sense of telling me or anything, because they didn't want me labeled. They tried to get me into special programs, but we were sort of between a rock and a hard place. We were too poor to afford special programs, but we were too rich to get assistance to be allowed into special programs.

And there weren't school special programs?

No, there was nothing. This was back in the early '70s in Los Angeles area. So I just had to do what I could. And some years the teacher would be good; some years the teacher would be bad. So my education would fluctuate.

SCHOOL EXPERIENCES: THE PRIMARY CHILDHOOD CONTEXT OF STIGMA

It is clear from the painful memories of many affected adults that children with NF1 frequently suffer through many years of sometimes excruciating teasing, taunts, and social assaults of various types and never tell their parents or other adults what they are experiencing. In addition to academic problems, many persons described how early physical symptoms constituted significant physical differences that other children noticed and censured them for, often resulting in feelings of shame and social alienation. It is difficult to distinguish neurological from physical, psychological, or social factors in their lack of academic and social achievement. Sarah pointed this up:

When you are sitting in a classroom you are not necessarily soaking up the information that is being put there. You are sitting there trying to hide your disfigurement, and hoping nobody will notice. You're thinking about what's been said to you at recess or on the way to class. You know, the person that knocked the books out of your hand, or whatever. Those are the things that obsess your mind, not what's being said in the classroom.

Randy hid a world of pain and depression after his first surgery, which he had after he was fourteen.

Some of my best friends knew I was having problems with tumors, and I was kind of ridiculed, saying I was going to turn into a tumor, and things like that. And then I got depressed. Some of my closest friends said, "We can't go out with you anymore because we're afraid if we touch you we're going to turn into a tumor." That hurt. But I just thought, "They don't understand."

Did you go home and tell your mom, or anyone?

Never did. I kept it all inside of me.

Subjects often said they had become "loners" as a result of their NF1:

As a teenager I think the NF alienated me from the other kids because of the growths. They may have had a fear that they were contagious. I didn't have a lot of close friends when I was growing up and I do think that had a lot to do with it. I would feel like saying, "You're not going to catch it; it's not contagious." People would still shy away.

Hyperactivity and the lack of coordination coupled to make Randy's childhood years difficult:

I try not to remember a lot of those things because it caused a lot of emotional stress for me back then. I always thought it was real difficult being a hyperactive child and wanting to be like everyone else. But with no one else wanting me around, because you run around; you're not sedate; you don't do the things that everyone else does, coupled with the fact that I wasn't really coordinated very well as a child. I think I was nine or ten before I learned how to ride a two-wheeled bike, so I was kind of left behind that way. So growing up, I spent a lot of time just watching television, reading comic books, fantasizing about what the world was going to be like.

And Elise:

Children can be very, very cruel, and there was never an adult who helped me. I didn't have friends, I was pegged from kindergarten. Teachers were irritated with me because of my learning disabilities, and I can remember being teased by the kids and being made fun of from K or first grade on.

Sharon's perception is that her parents did not understand her difficulties as a child and adolescent:

Looking back, I think that some of it was that I was so unhappy, but my folks treated it as a discipline problem, that I was being naughty because I wasn't doing well in school. Bless their hearts, they did the best they could, but it never occurred to them that maybe they should let me talk to someone, that I was unhappy because I had that large tumor on my leg, or that I was unhappy because I was taller and fatter than anyone else, or that I wasn't allowed to wear makeup, or that I wore glasses.

Because of all of these things I was miserable. Maybe I had some feelings that I needed to share with someone. Today I think people are more educated to understand that sometimes you need to talk to somebody, that sometimes you need to get help. It isn't just that you are going through a stage.

Frequent surgeries caused several subjects to miss school and sometimes exacerbated the problems of already faltering educational careers. Rachel, a very well-educated and philosophical women who contributed greatly to my personal understanding of the effects of NF1, did not have learning disorders, yet her memories of her school years were also very negative. She presented this analysis of her school problems:

It was very, very difficult growing up. And energy levels were always weak. Socially, I was a pariah in high school. I mean, I never had dates. I never had a lot of friends. I was a pretty lonely kid. And, it didn't matter what good grades you got. Good grades don't mean anything when you eat lunch alone.

You said you were a pariah? How do you mean that?

I felt very, very isolated from my peers. I missed lots of school because of the surgeries. And, when I finally returned to school, I didn't know anything. I mean, I knew the answers to the questions, but I didn't share in little secrets. I didn't know what was happening in the school. I wasn't socially adapted. I had a hard time making friends, because you make friends and then you go back into the hospital. And, all I ever did was read.

There were definitely times when I used to think, why am I alive? You know, I used to sort of contemplate killing myself when I was an adolescent, but I never could figure out how you do it. I just thought about it a lot. Because I couldn't see going on living with the pain. And, I was really lonely and I was really ugly. And, I thought who would ever love this ugly body? Adolescence is no fun anyway. Even with a normal, healthy, well developed, balanced child, adolescence turns them into monsters. And even more so with a genetically challenged childhood. It was really rough going.

Undressing for physical education stands out in the memories of many women in the general population as being an awkward and embarrassing activity. For those with visible symptoms of NF1 it constituted a particularly distressing ritual. A number of women talked about painful memories of undressing in physical education class and how their tumors were made visible to the world. Said Sharon:

My worst experiences were when I had to shower at school. The tumor on my leg got larger and larger. And, in fact, when I was in high school it was enormous. It got to be this huge thing just hanging down and that was the thing that people used to look at and comment about. At that point in life, when you're a young person, when you're a teenager, you're very aware of things that make you different. And so consequently, I actually hated gym because you know somebody's going to look at them. The kids said, "What are those things on your legs?" And I'd say, "Well, you know, they're called von Recklinghausen and they're hereditary. You can't catch anything from me and they're not going to hurt me." And you know, you try to make light of it but at the same time you're aware that they're really unattractive.

Sarah has often played "victim," a role that she feels originated in her early school days:

When you are told that you are ugly, stupid, and are not worth anything and you're not invited to play games with people and so on, it tends to make you feel not so great. I had the worst case so that left me vulnerable both at school and at home. I hid my vulnerability in the way that I carried myself differently.

Why did you carry yourself differently?

My vulnerability. My head would be down. I was terrified of people most of the time. I figured that when they spoke to me they would say something nasty or not say anything at all. Which of course, reinforced more vulnerability and more sadness. I think as a result of that, I believe that victimization is a learned role. I also believe that once you have been victimized in a learned role, it has a tendency to self-perpetuate and because you get deeper and deeper into that, there is no reference point for yourself as a person who is not a victim. If I am treated normally, I might tend not to believe it. At one point it was hard for me to understand why anyone would want to be nice to me. I probably felt that I didn't deserve to be treated better.

Three men talked about their special difficulties with sports. The fact that they were unable to engage in the typical round of sports activities was a source of shame to them.

Painful harassment factored into many of the subjects' lives, and individuals developed different coping styles. Harry described a social career marked by the taunting of his peers and adoption by "rough" protectors:

My social life was not very good at all. They'd always make fun of me. Give me a bad time. Push me around. I was different. I couldn't keep up. I looked different. I had a bigger head, droopy eye. Obviously, I couldn't do what they do. Deformed, I guess. I don't like that word, but this was true.

How did you deal with that?

It hurt, but I learned to adjust to it and grow up with it. Actually, some very weird things happened. I've got to be honest about it. When I started seventh grade in southern California, I went to junior high school, and I was obviously different. I didn't know much at the time. Streetwise, not much. Peoplewise, not much. I can remember being stabbed in the back by a kid in school. My father would never go to this school and do anything about it. But what ended up happening, this group of Mexican guys; at that time we called them Chicanos, now they're Brown Berets, they adopted me. And they started teaching me street things.

In junior high some kids hit me across the head with a hammer. That was pretty painful. But the next day, things were different. The guy that done it got roughed up. The rougher elements of the school adopted me as their buddy. That went on and then I got involved in the Air Force base where my father was stationed. So then again, the rougher elements of the society adopted me. Tried to teach me things like how to survive. Then eventually I ended up with the Hells Angels [motorcycle club]. I used to run around with them. But I never got in trouble. I just went to parties with them, drank with them. No drugs. Only alcohol. Then in high school, the athletes started to take me on as their buddy. So I went there as a manager. I'd pass out towels to them, help them fix their equipment. I was part of the clique then.

Why did some of these "rougher elements," as you call them, adopt you?

I don't know. Maybe because I was an outcast like they were.

Several persons commented on teachers who made special efforts to help them through school. Said Norita:

I had a lot of wonderful people that pushed me. And when I'm talking about pushing, now that I picture it, it was like I'm dropping dead on the ground. My teachers pushed me to the point that they didn't give me any breaks. One teacher pushed me and made me read every day, and made me read aloud, until I could pass. I mean, every single day after school for two hours she made do this. And I used to think, "That's so mean of them." And now I look back and I think, "If it wouldn't have been for them, I would not be here because they were so proud of every little accomplishment that I made."

Norita's teachers spent so much time with her that she did not want to fail them. Now some fifteen years later she has stayed in contact with some of these teachers.

College Experiences

Twenty-one of the twenty-eight adults who had learning disabilities went on to college, most often two-year community colleges. Their problems in learning continued to plague them there and eleven gave up in frustration. However, five of the twenty-one who went on completed four-year colleges with bachelor's degrees and two went on for master's degrees. Many commented on the difficulties of their college experiences. For example, Terry said:

I flunked my placement tests. If it had been verbal I probably would have done wonderful. I can't learn under pressure. I always did my book reports six months ahead of time. If the questions in the test were worded the same way the lectures were given, I did fine. If they were worded differently, I had trouble understanding what they wanted. I would have some teachers give me an essay test and I figured out how to go up and say, "Could you rephrase this one?" "Can you tell me this a different way?" Or, "What do you mean by this? I don't understand it." If they rephrased it the exact same way as in the lecture I would get it. With multiple choice tests I would have a very, very hard time. I would have to read and reread the question six and seven times in order to put it into a way I could understand it.

Three persons who graduated from universities described their careful interspersing of surgeries with the demands of school. Their persistence and determination were apparent in their accounts. Benjamin recounted:

One tumor that was removed from my thigh was about the size of a softball, and then six months later it grew back. It was funny because I was teaching classes on a fellowship. I gave all my students finals a day early, and then on the following Monday night of the week I was supposed to graduate I went into the hospital, had surgery on Tuesday, got out of the hospital on Wednesday, drove to Los Angeles and picked up my parents on Thursday and walked through graduation ceremonies on Friday with stitches in my left leg.

Rudy timed the removal of an eye during the midterm break of his final year of college so that the surgery did not cause him to miss classes. He then scheduled additional surgery on his eyelid for spring and summer.

Scheduling surgery for break time was insufficient help for Rachel because her energy flagged in graduate school when she had numerous hip surgeries.

I realized that I just didn't have the energy to go on for a doctorate. I was in the midst of having some surgeries on my hips when I was in graduate school. Every nine weeks, I'd have yet another surgery during quarter break. I didn't tell anyone. Because you're not supposed to tell anyone you have NF. You're supposed to just slog along with it. They were very painful recoveries and were long and I didn't do as well in school as I should have. I was sleeping a lot.

Did your advisor know about the surgeries?

Well actually, my advisor did. I had a research assistantship when I was in graduate school and the man I was working with knew. He knew that I was going into the hospital a lot. Also he would often find me sleeping in the library, I was just so exhausted. But, I had a full research assistantship when I was there. It was just crazy. This is just the kind of person I am. I just kept working.

The importance of economic resources for the educational career was pointed up by the experience of Richard, a man who came from a family with considerable economic and social resources. Richard's wife described her husband's passage through school and success in business.

He did dreadfully in school, but he got "gentleman's C's." For high school he went east and finally finished at an exclusive prep school in New Jersey. It's hard to fail out of those places. Even today you have to do something gross on the citizenship level. It's very hard to be cast out of a place like that, unless you're a total flake. Afterwards, he went to two private colleges but never finished. He entered the family business and sales after that. He doesn't talk about school at all. He talks about his college roommates; they're still very close friends. But he doesn't talk much about school experiences. I think he learned to compensate in his personality. He's just the nicest, warmest, most gentlemanly person I've ever encountered. But his children [with NF1] who have the same disabilities have had trouble from day one because Richard never dealt with them squarely.

This case, while the only one in the sample, suggests that particularly well favored families who are able to send their children to private schools and colleges and provide a protected work environment may be able to comfortably cushion the necessary challenges of life for them. These families are not ordinarily seen at NF support groups, nor do they in any way publicize their condition.

Contemporary Life

Learning disabilities continue to be a significant hindrance to many subjects. Even the brightest individuals often feel slow and stupid. Diverse kinds of problems that subjects experienced in childhood continue to plague them as adults. Most had concerns with reading, and difficulties span comprehension, spelling, and pronunciation. For instance, Carrie said:

If I start to read, I won't remember what I've read from the top to the bottom of it. By the time I get to the bottom, I don't know what they said on top. So, I don't read. It gets to be frustrating. Like I got my little grandson, Ray, into a book club. I read his books, the Fraggle books, because I like them. But I can't remember what happened by the end of the book. And those are *his* books. So if I can't remember that stuff, why should I bother to sit down and try to read anything else that won't stay with me anyhow? So, I just gave it up. Now I don't get so frustrated, because I just don't read, so that cures that.

Cecilia said:

I always got good grades but there are certain words that if I see them, I can't pronounce them. And I used to get laughed at because I pronounced words funny. But it's like I see the word but I can't make my brain or mouth say it.

Others talked about problems with the management of finances and organization at home and work. Jim said:

What happens since I'm not good at financing or figuring out things is that my aunt helps me and is like a financial advisor. She keeps the finances balanced so I won't overspend for that month or I'll end up having nothing for next month.

At least ten persons commented on their lack of coordination, or distinguishing left from right. Elise described an incident that had happened the week before:

A woman of my age, in her forties, came in the store with her parents and she asked where a certain department was. I said, "Oh, it's to the left," and then I pointed to the right. I looked at her and I saw that she had NF. I said, "I have no sense of direction." And the woman said, "I don't have a sense of direction either." I said to her, "I have NF and I think maybe you do, too." She said, "Yes," that she did. And she said, "You know, everybody I've met with NF shares this problem. They don't have a sense of direction."

My conversations with adults reflected the fact that despite whatever visible tumors or other symptoms subjects experienced, in most cases where learning disabilities and associated cognitive symptoms existed these were emphasized as being instrumental in causing long-remembered painful educational experiences. Likewise, they were cited as the chief obstacles in obtaining satisfying jobs that paid well enough to sustain a comfortable lifestyle.

6

Getting and Keeping a Job

In speaking of the job that she desperately hated, Sarah observed:

People who look different, people with disabilities, often do get treated pretty much like The Elephant Man. You may not literally end up in a freak show, but on one level or another there are many equivalents of freak shows, many dead-end jobs. And when you think about it, the person with the dead-end job is the one you hand the trash work that you don't want to be bothered with. *You* don't have time to do it. *You* don't get paid to do *those things. You* get paid to do more valuable work. And the person in the dead-end job also stays in the dead-end job because there is nowhere to move and there are no opportunities. It's kind of the equivalent of a freak show in itself.

The Elephant Man and the freak show have become metaphors for the discrimination and tortuous boredom of the low-level job in which Sarah, a bright, articulate and creative person, felt she was unfairly trapped.

All of the subjects chronicled their work experiences during the course of the interviews. Their occupations spanned an enormous range: corporate executive; nursery, primary, intermediate, and high school teacher; librarian; nutritionist; college counselor; nurse and nurse's aide; banker; receptionist; clerk; security officer; salesperson; factory worker; truck driver; electronic technician; supply clerk; waitress; homemaker; maintenance mechanic; and retired army officer. Nine persons were on short-term or long-term disability status related to their NF1. Specifically, occupations fell into the following categories: professional/managerial (14), service (waitress, fast food, sales, nurse's aide) (8), laborer, factory, truck driver (8), homemaker (4), retired from professional or clerical work (3), disability (9).

Twenty-six (just under half of the adults) reported that their NF1 condition had intruded significantly upon their aspirations, vocational options, and/or actual work experiences. In some cases their condition severely compromised their health and made work difficult or even impossible. Three men, one in his fifties and two in their thirties, who had previously been working, died of NF1-related causes during the research. Nine persons (five men and four women) were living on disability benefits at the time of interviewing. Two persons were recovering from spinal or leg surgery, three persons were totally incapacitated from spinal tumors or problems subsequent to surgery and were on long-term, permanent disability. Four persons were on disability for psychological reasons (depression, pain medication addiction, and/or general incapacity caused by severe learning disorders). These cases of death and disabilities represent the severest examples of physically debilitating conditions in the sample.

Eight of the twenty-six described how, in less severe ways, their NF had limited their choices or actually determined their being saddled with dissatisfying and ill-paying jobs. In two cases this was reported to be due completely to learning disorders, and in six to a combination of physical problems and learning disorders.

Every one of the twenty-six persons who described problems had learning disorders with the exception of two persons who were forced to go on disability assistance because of spinal tumors and their consequences. Yet of the approximately one-half who reported no consequences of NF1 for their employment careers, four also reported learning disorders while in school. These persons either received job training in community colleges and went on to work in areas of their specific competencies, or went right from high school without problems into long-term employment. About half of the subjects reporting no employment difficulties have at least some facial or other visible tumors. These persons represent many different educational and family backgrounds. However what most of them share are assertive personalities, determination and persistence, and good organizational skills.

Many subjects feel they are triply disadvantaged for employment because of their appearance, medical problems, and learning disabilities, which preclude their being able to manage many types of work. Numerous persons of the twenty-six who reported intrusion of the NF1 on their work careers spoke eloquently and poignantly about the ways in which NF has impinged upon or actually determined their employment opportunities and careers. I repeat here the words of Peter, a bright, highly analytic, articulate thirty-two-year-old factory worker who earned a living far beneath his capacities. He characterized the global nature of his problems:

I've always worked in factories and taken these low paying jobs—less educated jobs that anybody can do. But, if I say that at the factory, I get bawled out 'cause not just *anybody* can work in a factory. Not just anybody can work in the freezing cold on an assembly line. They smash their fingers and all. I know I take the vocational tests and I'm supposed to be like a doctor or somebody who cares, like the medical profession or a priest or something like that. I talk funny. I don't know how to talk. I can't sell cars or work in an office. I don't want to be fifty years old and have to work in this factory. When I thought of getting other jobs, I always feared that people would notice this skin disease, and, yet, they probably wouldn't.

Peter believes the psychological ramifications of NF1 are more serious than the physical effects.

I keep going back to the physical versus the mental of NF. The mental is more deeper than the physical effect of the disease—at least it is in our family. Do the people that you run into have mental blocks?

What do you mean "mental blocks"?

Like me, like they think they can't do this; they can't do that. They think they are held down because of the way they look. Like my mother can't go out in public. She says it's too long of a drive to town but I know that it's just that she doesn't want to go out in public. It's sad. I hope I don't get so bad that I look like that.

And Robbie:

Because of my dyslexia and spiral vision, I reverse numbers and letters, particularly numbers. Schooling was difficult for me. I could do it, but I had to work very hard to make fair grades and understand things. They tried to train me for banking. I took the test and halfway through correcting it, they gave up because I did so badly. My typing is abominable. When I spell, I can't tell if a word is wrong, and I can't stop and look up every single word in the dictionary. My eye-hand coordination is bad and I just cannot get up speed.

Societal stigma is highlighted as a major problem affected persons face in initial hurdles of employment and also afterward in keeping their jobs. Seven persons talked about being discriminated against in hiring because of facial tumors or skeletal differences. They clearly blamed the stigma around their appearance for their hiring difficulties. Pam, who has many tumors on her face, has been turned down many times for office work or other jobs for which she felt she was very qualified but where she would be in public view. "They want to make sure they don't have someone that other people would think was an eyesore working in front of the public. I think that has a lot to do with how I do in job interviews. I think that that has a big effect on the interviewer." Her numerous tumors may account for why Pam was not hired as an executive secretary, a position she had sought for months. Despite her qualifications and excellent references she did not get the job and feels that having facial growths had affected her chances. Pam said:

People are what they are and you don't want to hire someone who looks different, with any kind of deformity. Perhaps, it makes others feel uncomfortable, a little helpless, that they don't know what to do with this person who is different. And perhaps it wouldn't project the proper corporate image.

Harry was also pessimistic about finding new employment. "I just know I'm not gonna get hired. I can go on all kinds of job interviews but I know what my chances are before I go. I see a lot of factors—I got deformities; I'm small. Short people have a tendency not to be hired anyhow."

And Maureen also expressed her discomfort at the response of her workmates to her NF1:

I feel very, very uncomfortable sometimes at the county hospital because the doctors I work with will be looking at my neck and my arms. They will be concentrating more on my body than on the things I am saying to them. I'm scared to leave my position in the hospital to go to the outside because of discrimination. I feel that maybe I'm somewhat protected, but I don't know. I would encounter discrimination if I went to private industry and tried to get a job. If I went for my physical exam I might be told that I can't be hired because I have too many health problems.

If you didn't have NF, would you want to move into something else?

I would, I would.

Maureen never identified in her accounts the irony that medically sophisticated health care providers in a hospital context should be so rudely curious about her appearance.

Jim recounted that his workmates sometimes say:

"What's wrong with you?" It makes me feel like I got the bubonic plague or something. At one job the people who worked with me thought it was something that was contagious. I told them it wasn't and the supervisor had to inform everyone in the department it was not a contagious type of thing that I have. They had to get the whole crew together in the cafeteria to explain to them what I have.

Because Victor has encountered difficulties when he has specified his special health condition, he no longer does so.

So I just don't state it. Matter of fact, my [affected] brother tried to get on where I had got on and they wouldn't hire him because I had to explain that my brother's got tumors in his bone. And he's got an "s" back [scoliosis], whatever that means. You know, it's too bad, because he's a real hard worker.

Several persons talked about discrimination based on a fear of the potential expense of their health plans. Said Jim:

They think, "We're going to put this person's application to one side and get someone else." That is another thing that happens to NF people. Employers think they are going to have to pay extra for the medical insurance, that every time we run to the doctor, the company's going to be affected.

Finding a company that provides adequate health insurance coverage was a concern for many subjects. For example, Clarise said:

I'm ready to scream. I've been looking for a different job for the last two years. I look in the newspaper and I feel like I'm wasting my time. If I call a company and I ask for the Personnel

Department and I ask if the company is hiring and they say, "We're just a small company; we're only about twenty people," I tell them, "Thanks anyway." I don't want to deal with any more small companies. I've had it with them. Low wages and rotten medical insurance, which is my chief concern.

Headaches, vision, spine and leg problems limited many subjects' work options and threatened daily work experiences. Jim said:

I'm stuck with this crappy guard company. I keep looking and I keep looking and I check with the State Employment Office and they say, "Go get your right eye fixed and we can get you work on electronic assembly." They think I can do electronic assembly work again, but I know I can't do it. And I have a cross vision that keeps me from doing any welding type of job. From what I hear at NF meetings, for people who have NF and are looking for jobs, it's like having the bubonic plague.

Formerly an executive secretary, Helen recounted:

I became so badly afflicted with migraine headaches that the doctor I was seeing said that I really needed to get out of that kind of work; it was too high pressure, too high stress. It probably contributed to the migraines. So now I have this awful, boring, low-paying job, but I don't have the headaches.

Before Lou went on disability because of her extreme scoliosis, she worked successfully as a bookkeeper at an autobody shop. Her back problem was not a hindrance there because she did not do strenuous tasks and could pace her sitting and walking. However, prior to that job she worked at a travel agency, "The travel agency job didn't work. I couldn't really sit that long because of my back, and I couldn't stand that long because my ankles swell up. It just was really too uncomfortable for me to do it."

Just as surgeries, doctor visits, and medication problems sometimes posed difficulties when subjects with NF1 were of school age, in adulthood they often created the hardship of repeatedly missing work. A person with NF1 may require flexible hours in order to accommodate visits to doctors.

The most frequent work-related problems were caused by learning disorders. Because learning disorders are invisible and often occur in bright articulate people, they may not be recognized as a legitimate disability. Repeated negative school experiences often heavily contributed to the development of poor self-images and a lack of self-confidence in confronting the work world and the challenges of employment. Subjects frequently did not present themselves in their best light nor instill confidence about their abilities in supervisors or workmates. Subjects reported that supervisors and peers sometimes think they are dumb and that their mental abilities are limited. Sarah angrily comments:

I feel really victimized. I get the leftovers, the real garbage work, real garbage. After two and a half years of this real garbage work, I feel inadequate doing anything *other* than garbage work—photocopying volumes of books—that kind of thing. There is no time to do anything that shows my competencies. That creates an atmosphere such that when I do something valid, no one believes I did it anyway, because they see me photocopying and hole-punching and being a go-for.

This seems to be a way to create a cheap labor force. If they don't consider learning disabilities to be a problem as long as you can do shit work, then they will always have someone to do the shit work.

And Michael:

Sometimes in a working situation I think it is the most disheartening when trying your very best but because of the fact that you have a learning disorder you find that it is hard for you to do what needs to be done. I could tell you of situations where I'm trying very, very hard and the boss comes over and says, "You dummy! You keep making the same mistake over and over. I can't believe you're so dumb." And you think, "Hey, I'm not that dumb. I'm doing the best that I can."

I was working for the phone company. I was trying my hardest to pull down calls and put calls together and get all the information and do everything. I was still slow and I made mistakes. I did about two-thirds of what the other operators were doing. Where I would feel I was just working up a sweat, just burning up the boards, I was handling maybe fifty calls an hour and the average for the board that day was sixty-five to seventy calls. And I am only doing fifty and I think I'm doing good. I've got this supervisor breathing down my neck saying, "Come on, do more. Can't you go faster? Do more." It was also a situation that I was always in trouble at the phone company, because of the fact that essentially I became a problem employee. I was slow and I made mistakes. So, subsequently, I was the one the supervisors always were looking at, whereas Betty or Judy or Sally or someone else down the board can sort of slow down for a little while, and kind of coast for awhile and not do as much work because they know the supervisor's not working on them as long as I'm on the board. Everybody's going to be watching Michael.

Several bright individuals who had had nonetheless miserable school records talked about their resultant poor self-images and generally discriminatory treatment at work. They described special talents that characteristically were not acknowledged by their supervisors or peers. For instance, Randy knows he has a talent for solving problems.

I find my job is most challenging when I'm trying to resolve where a lost receipt is, or why this receipt was applied to this account, or what's wrong with it. I don't like to sound arrogant or self-centered or conceited, but I know that in my unit there are only two people, and one of them is the supervisor, who know more on the computer screens than I do. About two months ago I came across a problem on an account that five people, counting me, had worked, and I was the only one that found the problem. If anything, my supervisor was mad why the problem hadn't been caught before, and then he took the credit for it, like he's done other times. In fact, I've taught him a lot of things on the job.

At least twelve of the twenty-six subjects reporting on the impact of NF1 on their work experiences and were employed at the time of interviewing, lived on the economic margins of society and could be categorized as the "working poor." The nine on disability were not counted in this number although the majority of them had also been impoverished when employed. These working poor depended on either low-paying jobs or part-time work. Most lived in geographic areas with a high cost of living, and tended to reside in very modest housing, in some cases mobile homes, and to have few consumer luxuries and essentially no discretionary funds. Rachel, who is a highly educated woman with several advanced degrees, feels that she lives on the economic brink. Said Rachel one day:

My real fear is to become like "Crazy Mary" who sits down in front of the bank on Market Street. I see her every morning, smoking cigarettes. I gave her some spare change one day and we started to chat. I do fear that I'm going to end up like that.

Why do you fear that?

Well, I work three-quarters time. I don't have a lot of money. I don't have much energy. What happens if the NF reacts again? This is the scenario: I lose my job, or I get laid off. I don't have the money to keep up my Harper Hospital payments. I can't get any other medical insurance because this is a preexisting condition. No other carrier is going to touch me. Basically, I am with Harper Hospital until they put me in the ground. This is the upshot.
I do worry that I'm going to be destitute, poor and old and sick and crazy. And who's going to take care of me? Nobody. It's real a fear that disabled people have. That edge, that little edge that keeps me *not* on the street and Crazy Mary *on* the street is really very fragile. It could break at any time. And I would be left there at the mercy of this great social service system. I know what goes on in county hospitals!

Pam, who identifies herself as one of the working poor, says, "We are essentially just a jump away from being homeless."

The self-perpetuating circularity of poverty in all aspects of life was illustrated by Jim, who barely subsisted on his low-paying hourly security guard wages. He lived in a modest mobile home he bought after selling his mother's home after her death and paying off his brother's half of the sale price. Jim talked to me about the major problems of his life, all seemingly connected in one way or another to his NF1. He repeatedly talked about his disenfranchisement from legitimate work options. He could not find employment other than guard work because of his many physical problems and limited reading abilities. Although Jim was a large and husky-appearing man, his torso was weakened by past tumors on his spine and an ongoing hernia problem so he could not physically manage warehousing or loading and delivery work. His loss of vision in one eye made operating heavy machinery impossible. His night work hours and grinding poverty precluded a social life and the rituals of dating. He could scarcely pay his rent and feed himself and his dog, his only companion.

Time and time again I heard accounts of serious economic consequences of NF1 for the lives of many persons. These consequences were dramatically illustrated throughout subjects' interviews, which often focused on their anxieties around employment and economic solvency.

DISCRIMINATION AND CIVIL RIGHTS

Many of the negative experiences recounted to me by subjects represented actions by employers and supervisors that have been illegal in the private sector since 1992. The civil rights of disabled persons, which includes those with genetic disabilities, are now protected by several federal laws and some state and municipal statutes. The Americans with Disabilities Act (ADA), passed in 1990, covers persons employed in the private sector in workplaces of fifteen or more employees and also in state and local governments. In California, state law lowers this number to five employees. The ADA offers antidiscrimination protection in employment, public services and accommodations, and telecommunications. The Rehabilitation Act of 1973 applies to persons working for the federal government or private sector workplaces that receive federal funds.

The ADA prohibits employers from using a job applicant's or employee's disability as a reason for not hiring or refusal of work opportunities if the person can perform the responsibilities of the job with or without reasonable accommodation. Likewise disabled employees must be given the same fringe benefits as other workers are given. The law prevents employers from making decisions about hiring based on probable costs to health, disability, life, and other insurance benefits. Further, workers cannot be given differential treatment because of a history of disability or because they may have a disabling condition at a future time.

Health insurance is a major concern of all Americans, and for those with special health conditions it may become the major consideration in employment. Employers may be loath to hire a person if they believe that person or their family members will be a major drain on their health insurance. The ADA prohibits employers from making decisions about hiring, retention, or advancement on the basis of possible medical costs for an employee or his/her family. The predictions that genetic testing has the possibility to offer information about an individual's health status that, if available to employers, could threaten their employment status must be taken seriously, and significant protection against this danger should be in place (Asch 1996).

The ADA, in stating that disabled workers who can fulfill their work responsibilities with (or without) "reasonable accommodation" extends protection to persons who have physical or cognitive limitations. Reasonable accommodation is a flexible concept that is interpreted on a case-by-case and place-by-place basis. Accommodation can vary from changes in the physical workplace to alterations in the style of training. For example, some persons may need a job coach and more time in the training period, or the adjustment and modification of examinations or training materials. Individuals with specific learning disabilities constitute the largest group requiring testing accommodations. Allowing additional time for completion of a test is a common accommodation for persons with learning disabilities but other accommodations also may be required (Brown 1994). Modifications of leave time and flexible schedules are also possibilities. However, the final performance standard should be the same for all employees.

Three persons recounted to me accommodations made for them that allowed them to work with more comfort. Benjamin was given a flexible schedule to accommodate surgeries and side affects of his medications. Terry also had a flexible time schedule because of her surgeries. Sharon felt her manager was extremely generous when, following her surgeries and rounds of chemotherapy, he brought a couch to the employees' lounge so she could rest in the afternoons. He also urged her to take as much time off as she needed. In fact, as a response to his generosity she tried to recover her energies as soon as possible, and often came into the office at 5:00 A.M., long before her workmates arrived.

The ADA wisely covers disabilities created by stigma and prejudice. Alleged discomfort of workmates or customers is no excuse for discrimination. Says Gostin:

The ADA expressly protects not only individuals who are actually disabled but also those who are "regarded" or perceived to be disabled. The law, therefore, does not objectively measure the actual abilities or disabilities of the person. Rather, it judges the discriminator through his own subjective perceptions, prejudices, and stereotypes. . . . It is the reaction of society, rather than the disability itself, which deprives the person of equal enjoyment of rights and services. (Gostin 1994:133, 134)

As a case in point, Gostin presents an example of a person with NF1:

A genetic condition which does not cause substantial impairment may not constitute a disability. If a person with neurofibromatosis, for example, has only mild changes in pigmentation she may not be disabled, but if she suffers from gross disfigurement she most assuredly would be protected under the ADA. (Gostin 1994:133)

Persons who feel their employment rights have been violated should complain to the United States Equal Employment Opportunity Commission within 290 days following an incident, and in California, to the Department of Fair Employment and Housing within 365 days. Most states have equivalent offices for complaints. Importantly, such complaints will put employers on notice that they cannot discriminate without consequences.

7

The Search for Intimacy

Many persons poignantly discussed the negative effects of their NF1 on dating and the development of sexually intimate relationships. Said Victor:

After we dated one time I said, "She's the one for me." A lot of it had to do with this little bird she had. It was kind of touching because it was a crippled little bird. I noticed that she loved this bird, so I thought that maybe she could relate to me and that maybe something could happen. I ain't saying I used that as an excuse for going with her, but I finally realized that people often do like things that are deformed or a little bit different. This was the first time I ever looked at things like this from a different perspective. Before that I always thought you had to be perfect or else you didn't fit in, like me.

And Jeraldine, in assessing the import of her NF1 on her sexual relationships:

My mother told me that God gave me my NF. Well, maybe God did give it to me. I like sex so much that if I didn't have this, then I'd be screwing my eyes out. So maybe God did give it to me to keep me from doing that.

The most moving accounts of life experiences centered on dating and sexual relationships. The foregoing chapters describe discrimination and interpersonal rejection often attributed to functional limitations around learning, reading, or other accomplishments necessary for school or work responsibilities. However, *none of the physical, physiological, or cognitive symptoms of NF1 can affect a person's ability to love.* Yet, societal pronouncements may discourage potential partners and engender attitudes of low self-worth in affected persons, contributing strongly to negative experiences in this most personal arena of life. The media vividly bombard us daily with societal prescriptions for "beauty" and health that are often linked to romantic success, despite the fact that relatively few persons in mainstream society are able to measure up to these prescriptions. Those persons who markedly differ from these cosmetic prescriptions may be overwhelmed by feelings of personal failure and inadequacy.

Most of the subjects have multiple small tumors and cafe-au-lait spots on various parts of their torsos. While not apparent with normal dress, nonetheless such bodily marks may seriously affect an individual's self-image, undermine their self-confidence, and inhibit their expectations and desires, particularly in matters of sexuality and the development and maintenance of sexual relationships. The barriers that both men and women face were made vivid to me when several men and women spontaneously offered to show me their abdomen or varied parts of their torso. In some cases the total skin surface was covered either by a solid sheet or a dense sprinkling of small tumors. In societies where physical difference is more easily tolerated these bodily features might not loom so large, but in a society such as ours, where rigid cosmetic prescriptions for beauty are so well advertised and reinforced, the challenges posed by the existence of numerous tumors, cafe-au-lait marks, or skeletal differences are daunting. Not only are affected persons made to feel inferior, but many potential partners are discouraged by their internalized values and by public and family opinion from pursuing relationships with persons who are physically different.

In the case of those whose symptoms were visible in their early years, their sensitivities about these symptoms often began in their teenage years or even younger when they felt shunned, rejected, and often isolated. Most did not date. Several persons related experiences of early rejection that created searing wounds on already weak self-images. Said Harry:

Never could date much in school, because didn't nobody want to be bothered with a "freak," as they put it then. That started when I was in the fifth grade. I think back, the deformities were starting to show up real bad then.

Did you date much in high school or in your young adult years?

No, never did.

Was it something that you thought about?

Oh, I thought about it a lot and I tried it a little, but you ask somebody out and they always tell you, "No," or they laugh at you. I didn't give up. It is hard, but I learned to adjust to it. People judge you by how you look, not by the person you are. If you've got these lumps and bumps on you, it is hard. Some people find it repulsive. They don't look at the personality. They say they might, but it doesn't work out that way.

Feeling estranged from normal adolescent dating activity burdened many subjects. Said Peter:

Up till nineteen I didn't think I could get anybody. I had crushes on girls, but I feared that they wouldn't want me because I had something wrong with me. I didn't date, nothing. That was what I went through in high school. I didn't want to get into social isolation. I didn't want to be sixty years old and not ever been laid. That's just the way it is. But, man, why be scarred with it mentally anymore than you already are? We're human, you know.

Carla also had a many difficulties with dating:

I feel very fortunate that I found my husband. When I was in school, there would be three of us eating. If two boys came over, they'd each take one girl on either side of me. I never dated at all in high school or college.

Many single persons related problems of social and sexual rejection that were ongoing in their thirties and forties. Sharon, who had tried several dating services, was certain that her moderately visible NF1 prevented what would begin as telephone relationships from developing further.

I talked to one man two or three times on the phone and he was great. Then, when we met for coffee, he said, "Oh, you must be Sharon. Sorry, I just have a few minutes. I have to go mow somebody's lawn." He sat down and absolutely choked down a cup of coffee and was out the door. On another dinner date I arranged through an ad, the guy only ordered soup, ate it in ten minutes and then got up and said, "I'm ending this relationship right now. I don't find you attractive." I said, "What relationship?" One of my theories is that men expect Cheryl Tiegs but they offer Don Rickles.

Ronald, an older bachelor who walks with a noticeable limp caused by leg and back tumors, finds he is too inhibited to attempt establishing new relationships. He feels that if he enters a singles bar or a social club the prevailing attitude is, "Who's interested in the 'gimp' comin' over here?" Ronald was discouraged by "uncomfortable feedback" about his appearance.

Adults dating in contemporary society, in contrast to the dating and premarital experiences of older subjects now married, find the normative expectations for achieving rapid intimacy in dating and courtship have brought concerns about physical symptoms to the fore. Premarital sexual relations are common and expected today. Few older persons in their dating years worried about being rejected offhand because of physical symptoms that were not likely to be exposed before marriage. The oldest married subjects (55+) had dated very little, often marrying their first boyfriend or girlfriend. In their dating period they typically were younger, had few or no visible symptoms, often did not know about their condition, and did not have sexual relations before marriage. Thus they did not have to confront the issues of physical or informational disclosure described to me with considerable anxiety by single persons. Said Isabelle, now in her late fifties:

I believed in romance, you know. I never associated sex with love because in the movies you just kissed and everything was wonderful. I never even thought about the sex part of it. I feel sorry for kids today; they have no innocence.

The contrast to this expression of older mores was very apparent in the accounts of dating given by younger subjects. Recounted Angela:

My first sexual experience ended with the man walking out because he thought my body was ugly. Now, what does that do to an eighteen-year-old? My questions were always sexuality questions. What does it mean to have NF and be aware of your sex? What does it mean when you're eighteen years old and all your contemporaries are discovering their bodies and physical pleasure with somebody else, and you don't? What does this do to your self-image? We are sexual beings. We are not meant to be celibate.

Many single women and men talked to me about their problems in exposing their tumors to partners with whom they expected to go to bed. Said Cecilia:

I said to him, "Listen, Jerry, if we're gonna sleep together we have to talk." I asked him all about his sexual history and told him about mine. Then I said, "I've something to tell you." And he said, "Don't you think I can feel you and see you? Don't you think that I know that there's something?" It kind of made me a little sad because I had been thinking I'd been hiding it. Then I thought, "But no, Cecilia, don't do this to yourself. If he's felt them and seen them on you and still wants to be intimate with you, then that must be saying something." But my first thought was, "I thought I was hiding it. How did he feel it; when did he feel it?" After we made love I said, "Oh, you're probably not gonna come back again." And he said, "Why do you say that?" And he did come back.

And Larry, a gay man:

In the beginning I couldn't ever understand why nothing happened with relationships. But after awhile I started feeling it was the NF. Sometimes I would meet someone, and they would have a bad reaction to my lesions. I've had people ask me to leave their beds, and others got up and left my place when they saw my body. Several years ago when the herpes scare first started, a lot of people thought I had herpes. Then, when AIDS came along some people thought I had AIDS. It can be very painful to have someone recoil from you like you're a leper. And that's happened. But if I was "normal," and I met someone with these things, I guess I would also be inhibited to get involved with them. So I don't feel hateful toward these people. They're reacting normally. It's a matter of finding that extra-special person where it doesn't matter.

I'm trying a new way now. I'm trying to be more reserved. I try to get to know someone very well before I get intimate with them. Maybe that might help. If they know me much better first, they might be more willing to accept me as I am.

At this point I do not have a sexual partner. I would like one. I'm not sure if I will have one again or not; I don't know. I'm trying to be open to it, but I'm not being so open that I think someone's going to drop out of the sky for me. I've pretty much made myself think that if I'm going to be single for the rest of my life, I'm going to make the best of it. I can't just wait around for someone wonderful coming my way. I have to make a life for myself and be open to a relationship. If it happens, fine. If not, I can still be happy.

Robbie thinks that without the NF lesions on his chest and back he would have stood a better chance of developing a relationship. He feels they will inhibit someone from wanting to get to know him better.

It does hurt realizing that I thought that these growths don't make a difference. But society and people say, "They do. They make a great deal of difference." And to have that underlined and thrown in your face for years—it just sort of digs it in. In a way you feel like an outcast. It stops me sometimes from pursuing someone because of fear of the rejection. So partially it's the NF, partially it's this fear of what would happen if I pursue something. Not wanting to have a bad experience again, because it does hurt. At first I could handle it—oh, this person is just shallow, but when for the umpteenth million time it seems to happen, I can only be teflon so much and have it bounce off. Sometimes it starts sticking. I am only human.

Randy, who is severely affected, finds it extremely difficult to tell anyone that:

"Yes, I may someday end up with lumps on my face." And asking them to want to be with me, that does bother me sometimes. When I'm in a relationship I get very scared that I may scare them off. And they do get very scared about those things. But I also know, and I once told somebody something that I guess I have to believe for myself, that you can run from relationships; you can run as far as you want, but sooner or later you're going to run into a wall, and when you do, you're going to have to stop running. And what I have to finally realize is that it's very scary for me to ask someone to be with me for ten years and believe I'm going to be alright. I may live until I'm eighty-five; I don't know. Somebody one time asked me, "Doesn't it scare you that you know you're going to die?" I said, "Everyone is going to die. Some of us just have a better knowledge of when than others do."

Norita told one man about her NF1 before they slept together and he did not seem bothered. One morning, however, he called angrily screaming at her, "You've given me NF! You've given me NF! I woke up this morning covered with brown bumps." Norita said, "I kept telling him that was impossible, but he was really mad and said he was leaving to see his doctor. Can you imagine this?"

Sarah did not inform her husband about her NF1 before they slept together. Nor does he know much about it today. Her low feelings of self-worth were reflected in this statement.

It has always made me extremely uncomfortable, wondering whether to say anything or not to say anything. Since most of the people who were supposed to be loving to me weren't accepting of it, I guess I am afraid that if he knows too much he will use it against me.

Actually, I've denied my sexual self, believing that I'm so ugly. Basically, how I feel is I'll be somebody's hole, and it won't matter what's attached. That sounds extremely crude, I'm sure, but it's indeed how I feel.

Some subjects described their forays into sexual encounters where they tried to hide their tumors by not undressing or in other ways. Jeraldine said that she was lucky that as a teenager she had a boyfriend.

I had a boyfriend at sixteen—from sixteen to twenty—who told me it didn't matter, he still loved me, and that he didn't care and these things didn't bother him. I would say it was a couple of months before I had let him pet me underneath my blouse. Anytime he tried to do it under my blouse, I was one of those that went, "No, no!" You know. [Laughing] And then finally one day, I said, "There's a reason why I haven't been letting you." And then he said, "Why?" And I remember, like I took a pillow, so that as soon as I opened my blouse, I could go like that [pressing the pillow to her chest] with the pillow. And then I told him what it was, that it was not contagious, that my mother has it, and it's hereditary. And then, I made the lights be out and he was very nice. "Oh, I love you; don't you know? I love you; it doesn't matter." And all that nice stuff.

Despite his assurances, Jeraldine was uncomfortable with being nude and would not have intercourse.

But I wouldn't feel comfortable getting naked for a long time. I still had those feelings of being ugly with my poor self-image inside. But at least I had somebody telling me, "I still love you."

When I came to California, I had a few one-night stands and again, I was able to get around it by not getting completely naked. Lots of times I wore a teddy or camisole, so it covered my trunk where most of them are, on my back and my belly. And, believe it or not, a lot of men aren't into getting you completely naked with the whole lovemaking behind it. I would make love with them once and manage without taking my clothes off. I always keep the lights off and I guess I always move around a lot, so that their hands don't get to touch every inch of me.

Lots of times, I'll close my eyes and I won't want to look at myself. That's the way *I* deal with it. I'd rather close my eyes and pretend like my body is smooth and regular, rather than to look down and see my NF tumors while the guys are kissing me and fondling me.

Happily, other women told of short- and long-term relationships in which boyfriends and lovers told them their physical marks did not matter. Angela had the good fortune of having a lover who accompanied her on a journey out of "denial" and "self-hate":

I went through a long period of denial. Denial that I had NF. Because of a sense of real self-hate that women and disabled women are taught, to hate themselves by this society. You open *Vogue* magazine. When you're a teenager, you open *Seventeen* magazine. And it's like a tyranny. I mean, my hips don't look like that. My shoulders don't look like that. I am hunched over and my body is ugly. And I had some devastating sexual experiences. Until I realized what I was voicing was self-hate, it was a slow journey learning to accept myself. I was fortunate because I had one lover who was wonderful on this journey of learning to accept my body. He told me that my back, with the cafe-au-lait marks, reminded him of a map of China—the way they come up through my shoulder and down most of my back. He said he could outline various parts of China on my back. And I really appreciated that. I'm sure most women with artistically beautiful bodies get told that they're beautiful all the time. But I was never told that. I was never told that I was beautiful. And that relationship, hearing those words, was the most important thing in the world to me. I was twenty-five then.

Carrie, a lesbian, said in her lively fashion:

Oh, none of my lovers didn't even care. It was like, "So what, no big thing," which was cool.

Did you explain it to them before you got intimate? Did you say anything?

Yeah. I let them know what it was. That I've got it; it's hereditary; and it's no big deal. It was always like, "Who cares? I'm just interested in you," which was cool. I've never had any problems with my lovers over it.

Norita talked about one boyfriend who was particularly supportive and positive around her condition.

I always do it in the dark, under the sheets. In the beginning I wouldn't let anybody see me naked.

How do you explain that?

I just tell them that I am very shy. With Joe, the first time he allowed it to be like that. Then, the next time, he wouldn't. Because people usually go away when I tell them about my NF, I went to my therapist to ask him whether to tell Joe or not to tell him. He said that it was better to tell him now. So after that I told him. I remember getting out of bed and putting my robe on and just walking away from him and telling him, "Well, you know, I have this." And he goes, "Is it contagious?" "No." He goes, "I don't care then." I cried, and he just held me in his arms. He was so kind, just very sweet. When we were first in bed I kept covering myself and he says, "No." And he got up and got a flashlight and he says, "Now, we're going to mark every single one [tumor]. I'm going to write a number on every single one that you have and we're going to keep a chart." At the time, it really bothered me, but then as time went by and he kept doing that, it stopped bothering me. I always thought, "He's not coming back. He's just like the others." But he kept calling me, asking me out. That has been nine months now since we have been dating.

Several persons buoyantly stated their philosophy that if a person did not accept them with their bodily marks then they did not want that person. For example, said Rosa:

Is this anything you were concerned about when you first got together with your husband?

No, that wasn't a problem with me. I was a little self-conscious because I do have the spots all over the trunk of my body. And I have quite a few scars, but the thing for me is that if you love me, then that's not going to make any difference. It's not going to matter to me and it's not going to matter to you. And if there's no love there, and if you really don't love me, then that's when it could make a difference. But I'm not a shy person. It's, "Take me as I am, or you know, don't bother." So I'm not really that self-conscious because it's just been something that I've had to deal with. I've dealt with it all my life, so, "Go with the flow."

While women, despite frequent negative experiences, persisted in the search for intimacy, a significant number of men retreated from dating or the pursuit of eventual marriage as early as the teenage years. These men cited their distaste for casual sex, concerns about having children, or economics. For example said Hal:

> The women that I do meet, they're single and they still want to have kids. And kids are out for me. There are some women out there who don't want kids, but are still a little on the wild side. And one nighters are definitely out for me. And especially now with the diseases. But I never liked one nighters, or just casual.
>
> *Was there ever a past relationship?*
>
> No. I've known that I'm not going to have kids. Since I'd like to get to know the women before I get serious with them, it's not going to go anywhere anyhow. So why play games? Why do something when you know it's going to end anyway?

This pattern of men's withdrawal in contrast to the behavior of women will be discussed in Chapter 9.

Subjects' accounts reflect a broad range of positive and negative experiences. It appears that many factors affected the nature and quality of subjects' dating and sexual experiences: gender; the expected social mores at the time of dating; actual visible physical symptoms, attitude, personality, and self-image of the subject; persistence; and simple fortune in where and when potential partners were encountered.

8

Marriage and Childbearing

Rachel embodied the feelings of many women in this study when she commented sadly:

All women have our share of problems. But, sexuality in NF is a real struggle. It's hard. It's hard in this society, in the baby boomer world where sensibilities are Madison Avenue and Ivy League. And, I don't look like the ideal. The world works on a "Noah principle" and it's very difficult to be alone. There's no joy, especially when I'm in a community where most of the women are married and are having babies or adopting them at a rapid, magnificent rate. It's very hard.

Issues of marriage and sexuality, and hard decisions about childbearing posed challenges for most of the participants in this research, both women and men alike.

The subjects related a broad diversity of marital experiences:

MARITAL STATUS	MEN	WOMEN
Currently married	10	20
Previously married	*0*	*4*
Single	12	12
Divorced	*2*	*5*
Never married	*10*	*7*
Never Married with children	*1*	*1*
Total	**22**	**32**

MARRIAGE

Of the fifty-four affected adults, thirty were currently married (twenty women and ten men). Of these, the majority described normatively functioning marriages. Two women reported (and were observed to have) unhappy problem-laden relationships that could have dissolved from day to day, and two men had long-term separations from their wives. Four currently married persons (all women) had had previous bad marriages. Seven (five women, two men) who were currently single had been divorced. Seventeen (seven women and ten men) had never been married. Of these never-marrieds, two have children.

While only seven of the thirty-two women had never been married (less than one-fourth of the total); ten of the twenty-two men, or almost one-half of the men, had never been married. The ages of these men represent a span almost as great as those who are married—from nineteen through the fifties. Only one married man was considerably older than the oldest unmarried male.

With the exception of the two very problematic marriages, marital relationships had not been seriously damaged by NF1-related symptoms or medical problems, although these may have posed challenges at varying periods. The impact of very visible tumors of some affected persons seems to have been adapted to and absorbed by their partners through the years. In the cases of the very visibly affected—typically aged fifty and above—when their marriages were conceived some twenty to forty years ago, there were few visible marks of NF1. Because courtships and marriages were ordinarily begun at earlier ages in the past, they predated the appearance of noticeable tumors, which often did not burgeon in women until during and after childbearing.

If symptoms were visible during the early years of the relationship, they were not considered significant by either spouse, and if the NF1 was diagnosed at the time, there was little known about it. Even when couples were told of its hereditary nature, neither they nor their doctors appear to have considered it a significant threat to their marriage or childbearing. Only in the two ongoing poor relationships and in those reported to have ended in divorce were tumors a serious issue. Said Faith:

I think I am more conscious of my NF because of Charlie. I guess I can't really blame him because it has been hard on him. He looks around him and sees other women who have smooth skin and you can't really blame him for being upset.

Has he ever said anything?

Oh, sometimes. My skin is so tender and sometimes he will come up and try to rub me and sometimes it does bother me, hurt me a little bit. He says, "I can't even touch you without it hurting." But there is one time I said something that I shouldn't. He latches onto anything like that. I said, "Maybe it's your fault that I got it." I read something once about the nerve endings and I thought maybe it was that he keeps me upset all the time. I said, "Maybe because you keep me upset all the time it causes it to come out more." Which is the truth. Now he says, "You said one time that I was the cause of it. Then I must have been the one that put it on my kids." One time he did say, "Whenever I rub your back it feels like a rubbing board." It hurts to hear him say something like that.

One visibly affected divorced woman, Grace, feels that her appearance factored into the problems of her marriage:

Do you think that NF1 was any particular part of the problems that led to divorce?

I feel it was. I don't know for sure. I mean, he never said it, but I feel it was. I felt really that I repulsed him. Once he turned away from me in bed, but at that time though, he'd been having an affair with another woman, and maybe he just rolled over thinking it was her, but it was me and he felt the difference.

As mentioned earlier, significant changes in the nature of dating and courtship have seriously impacted those persons currently in search of marriage. In past years, dating was much less explicitly sexual in nature. Also, premarital communication was not as candid in its examination of potential issues and problems to be encountered in marriage. In addition, in the pretelevision years, and even in the early period of television, the daily influence of the media was much less, and media messages were not so specific, vivid, and comprehensive in defining and reinforcing cosmetic prescriptions for beauty and health. These factors precluded many of the problems for older subjects that now affect single subjects, both never-married and divorced. For example, said Theresa, a woman in her late fifties, who was moderately visibly affected at the time of interviewing:

We weren't quite as open twenty-five years ago as we are since the sexual revolution. [Laughing] When my husband and I got married, I remember saying to him something like, "I've got these bumps." At the time, when he and I first went together, I didn't have any on my face and I didn't have any on my hands. I told him, "I want you to know that I have these things on my body and they are called von Recklinghausen; they are hereditary and it's possible that if we ever have any kids, that they would get the same bumps." And he assured me that was not a problem to him.

Was your husband the first man that you dated?

Seriously, yes. But you know what, with my husband? The day I met my husband, I really liked him. I was fifteen years old and it's like an instant attraction because he was kind and he's nice and I really liked him. And I was not afraid to be with him. But I was very afraid of boys. Like I was fine just talking, but if I was asked for a date it was always, "No." I didn't want to go out because I was afraid. I don't know what I was afraid of, looking back.

Three previously divorced and now single persons stated that they believe their physical symptoms would preclude another relationship. For example, I asked Pam, a very visibly affected woman:

Do you have any image as to what this issue would have done if your marriage had continued? Would your ex-husband have tolerated this? Would it bother him?

I would think he probably, yes, would have tolerated it. But as far as a future marriage or entanglement—I would worry, totally, because no man could accept the way I look now. This is perhaps a total irrational thought, but it's there.

Even two women who would be considered beautiful by American cosmetic standards expressed their fears about the possibility of remarriage if something happened to their husbands. Said one of these:

I'd be afraid that I might get these tumors all over my face and that if I had to I couldn't find anyone else that would want me like this. My husband jokes with me and says, "Oh, I'll always love you. I may have to put a bag over your head, but I'll always love you." But maybe I couldn't find anyone else to love me.

The persons who were divorced recount often acrimonious former marriages, highly traumatic and tragic in their effects on spouses and children. Several of those divorced recounted that they had been unhappy as teenagers and young adults and had been precipitously driven into bad relationships because of their poor self-images and low expectations for finding an appropriate partner. Their initial meetings with their former spouses were typically inauspicious. For example, said one woman: "I met him at a friend's house when I was twenty-two and he was nineteen. I think I hung out with him at first because I was so lonely, and I felt so ugly and awkward. Having somebody was better than having nobody."

Health problems related to NF1 sometimes contributed to wrecking even positive relationships. Benjamin recounted:

My marriage was pretty bad. I was on drugs for pain most of the time, and I was having surgeries. I figured I was married to her for almost eight years and I had thirteen surgeries during those eight years.

Was she supportive of you?

She was very supportive at first. She was there for me, but it was finally too much for her. I don't want to get married again. I'm afraid things would start going wrong again and that I'd become a burden on the person. It scares me.

Harry also did not think he would ever remarry. His condition has worsened since his divorce. "No, I don't think I'll ever marry again. I think it's too much trouble. The mom of Cleo, the girlfriend I have now, doesn't want her to marry me cause she's afraid that Cleo will do the same thing my ex-wife did if I get worse—just walk out. And I can't do as much for myself now as I did then."

CHILDBEARING

For those persons who carry a problematic dominant genetic condition and face a fifty-fifty chance in every birth of passing on this condition, issues around childbearing and pregnancy may be agonizing and overwhelming. The burgeoning literature on decisions about childbearing in the presence of genetic disorders tends to focus on issues surrounding prenatal testing and diagnosis and attitudes toward selective abortion. Very little in the literature has questioned subjects retrospectively about how in the past before such tests existed or were perfected they decided to have children while knowing they carried a dominant condition.

During the interviewing period for this study genetic marker testing was available, but could only be used in situations where there were two or more already known to be affected family members available for comparison testing. Currently prenatal testing using *in vitro* Transcription/Translation assay can identify causative mutations in 70 percent of cases. Prenatal testing through amniotic fluids or chorionic villi sampling will pick up NF1 mutations with 100 percent accuracy, if an affected parent can also be tested (Heim et al. 1995). Nonetheless, a positive test will not disclose which of the many possible symptoms of NF1 a baby may exhibit nor give an indication of what he or she may expect as an adult. The severity of the case of a parent does not reveal the severity of what his or her child's case might be. While a number of centers across the country have been able to do prenatal testing for several years, few persons have opted for the procedure.

Benjamin et al. (1993) in their study of eighty-one subjects in the northwest of England investigated reproductive decisions of fifty-six NF1-affected patients and twenty-five unaffected parents of affected children. They found that 44 percent of the thirty-two subjects at risk for having a child with NF1 who knew this before having their family said that it had influenced their reproductive choices. Those who reported no influence said this was because they knew little about the condition or because they had a great desire for children. Yet most of those who knew about the risk did not refrain from having children, a major complicating factor being the variability in presentation. A total of 34 percent of the twenty-nine who had no prior knowledge of NF1 reported that it would have influenced their reproductive plans if they had known. And 41 percent of the twenty-nine subjects who were still considering children wished to have a prenatal diagnosis in a future pregnancy, but only three of these reported that they would terminate an affected pregnancy (Benjamin et al. 1993:567, 571–572).

In my sample, issues around pregnancy and childbearing posed a number of serious dilemmas, particularly for affected women subjects. Many feared the possibility of exacerbating the visibility or severity of their condition as well as passing on NF1 to any children they might have. Very few were directed to genetic counselors to assist them in decision making. It is noteworthy that married, divorced, and single women and men were not hesitant to talk about the knotty issues of childbearing as they thought about them currently or remembered them at their times of decisions.

About half of twenty-seven in this study who had children stated that they either did not know that they had NF1 at the time they conceived, were not told that it was hereditary, or were told it would not be a serious condition to pass on. In Florence's case, her doctor dismissed her tumors: " 'Oh, not to worry,' and so I never thought anything more about it. He did not tell me that it was genetic."

Four women were initially diagnosed during their pregnancies or at childbirth, some by doctors who chided them for being pregnant with the condition. Said one woman: "He took one look at me and immediately said, 'You've got neurofibromatosis and you shouldn't be pregnant.' Well, I was four months pregnant by then. What could I do?"

Ten subjects were told they had NF1 but were given minimal information and they were not told that the condition was hereditary. Lily told me, "When I got pregnant we didn't dream that it could be passed on." In four cases subjects reported they were told that because they did not have a severe case, even if their child might inherit the condition there would be no reason to worry.

However, some accounts reflect that although some women may not have been told that the condition was hereditary, they had an inkling that it might be. Several others knew there was the possibility. Ambiguity may have characterized the issue of childbearing, but clearly the desire to have children was the chief deciding factor. For example, said Laura:

No. I did not know that it was hereditary.

Had you thought about it?

I thought that maybe one of the kids would have it but I really didn't feel it deep enough to say, "Let's not have children." Because we did have children. And these children were planned.

Rhoda matter-of-factly stated she forgot about her diagnosis by the time of her marriage. "It was seven years or so until I met and married my husband. I just didn't think anything about it."

A few women reported that doctors gave them extreme and "scary" predictions but even these did not convince them not to have children. For example, Marilee, who knew she had inherited NF1 from her mother, was sent to a geneticist by her regular doctor when she was pregnant with her second child.

That was my first experience with a geneticist. I had never even thought of going to a geneticist. I think now that it is wise. I probably should have been going to one for a long, long time. He talked with me and told me that it was a fifty-fifty chance and that there were these things that we needed to worry about in a child, things to watch for. They were real scary. He told me about the big stuff like the growths on the brain and the spinal cord and the eyes and the stuff that would really inhibit, that would really be a health challenge for a kid. That concerned me but it didn't make me feel like not having any more children. The only reason that Lindsey was my last child was because of her prematurity. I had preeclampsia and the doctor said, "You are definitely not a pregnant person. You should probably never, ever get pregnant again. The next time, you might die."

For others the "scariness" made its impact. Jody's geneticist told her:

"You are probably playing with fire. You've got at least a fifty-fifty chance of passing it on again, plus the fact that you may do further damage to your own health." And before Jay and I even got out to the car, we basically looked at each other, and said, "This is ridiculous. It would be foolish to even try it again." And so that's when we began to pursue the idea of thinking about an adoption as opposed to not having any more children. But we basically decided then, it's not worth risking my health, or possibly passing it to another child, who may not even survive a pregnancy. It is not worth it. So we didn't even think twice about going ahead with it any further.

I remember seeing a woman that I sat next to at one of the big NF meetings who had small little ones, you know, like little pock marks all over her face, and all over her neck. And I remember her telling me that she had four or five children and two of them had NF. She knew after the first child that she had NF, and she continued to get pregnant and have more children. And I remember being bold enough to ask her why she continued to have children and she said because her husband wanted more children. I really felt very sorry for her, because she knew that she was getting progressively worse each time. And I thought that was kind of sad that she either didn't have a husband that was understanding enough or that she didn't tell him or she wasn't willing to go do something about it. We both felt very strongly that it wasn't worth risking my health or possibly passing it on.

Although most persons who saw geneticists reported them to be neutral even when giving negative information, several recounted other doctors and even a few geneticists who were zealous in recommending against conception. Said Claire resentfully, "The doctor advised me 100 percent to get my tubes tied. I did that but I felt like I was giving up my womanhood. I felt a lot had been taken away when I had my tubes tied."

Elise wryly told me about the diverse opinions she had received from a variety of doctors. Initially she saw a neurologist to learn the specific ramifications her NF1 might have on childbearing.

He was incredibly rude. At the end of my appointment he made a big deal of moving his sleeve up and looking at his watch and putting his arm down and then he said, "You just wasted forty-five minutes of my time. You just go out and have all the babies you want to have." His anger was that he had patients with real difficulties with NF and that my case was so insignificant that I had wasted his time. But why didn't he tell me something like, "You're one of the lucky ones, but we can't guarantee that your children will be. If you do decide to have children, and they do, in fact, have it, there is no way that we can tell to what degree they will have it."

She and her husband proceeded to have a son who was born with NF1 and Elise next consulted a geneticist who told her:

"There is such a variability within the disorder that you could have a baby that would live their whole life probably like anyone else. The NF can be so mild it goes undiagnosed their whole life, or at the other end of the spectrum, you quite literally could give birth to a monster." And he said, "What I mean by monster is that you could give birth to a baby that looks like a Hollywood make up artist had gotten hold of the child for a horror movie." I don't know what comes to mind if somebody would say that to you. I can get no visual picture at all. Maybe I haven't seen enough horror movies. But, that to me was being overly dramatic and very cruel because there was that part of me that knew that there was no way on earth I was going to give birth to a monster. However, if he had shown me a picture of a baby with tumors all over its body or somebody who had lost an eye because of an optic glioma, or any number of things that you and I have now seen, that's something I could have looked at and said, "Okay, this will help me make my decision." But that isn't what I was told. Instead I was told that I could give birth to a monster.

This grim message did not discourage her. When Elise was pregnant the second time, she consulted another neurologist who "read her the Riot Act."

He said that had he been my doctor while I was growing up, he would have seen to it that I never had children. He said, "I would have scared you so badly, you wouldn't consider having children." And he said that he had case histories that would turn me white over night if I ever wanted to read them. He said I could have a severely retarded child, a child born with wasted limbs or huge limbs. "You can have a child born blind; you can have a child that is just nothing but a mass of tumors." Later this doctor did a complete reversal and apologized profusely for everything he had said at that first meeting. He said, "You have a beautiful child. I would have made a drastic mistake by encouraging you not to have children. Everything I told you was based purely on textbook knowledge, not on real people. It's the type of stuff they teach you in medical school to scare you."

How did he come to that?

I don't know. I think after we left, he probably realized how he must have sounded to me. He just let this twenty-eight-year-old woman in her sixth or seventh month of pregnancy have it. He was very, very tactless with everything he said to me. I think he wanted a chance to apologize and maybe try to right some of the damage he felt he may have done. And he said he very much wanted to be there when this baby was born and for me not to worry.

In three cases subjects who had one child stated their children were "accidents," and once conceived, they did not consider abortion. Said Michael:

We were newlyweds, three years married, and we thought that we had our whole lives ahead of us to worry about kids and NF and all that. We were more concerned with just living from day to day and going camping and going here and there. Then, all of a sudden, she became pregnant and it was like, "Whoa, I guess it's time to kind of like close the barn door after the horses have gotten out." But then we started to think about what we had done and what we had to do in the future.

And Benjamin:

I just thought my mom has it, and I got it. It's the simplistic way I thought about it. My wife got pregnant by accident even. I had genetic tests on me and the doctors told me there was no way possible I'd get my wife pregnant. Low sperm count, everything—everything against me to be able to father a child, but I was able for some reason, and by accident she got pregnant.

Did you want to have children?

I did. But I've even had bishops in my church tell me not to have any children because of the circumstances.

Several mothers talked about their guilt in having had children. However, the births were also recognized as blessings that would always be precious despite the hazards. Said Jodie:

I've gone through a lot of guilt over my daughter even though I didn't know when she was born that I had NF. Except for the scoliosis, so far she doesn't look that different. We're hoping that as mine's mild, hers will be mild. So maybe we haven't given her something that terrible. But we wouldn't try it again. If you ask me now if we'd known about NF and my having it before we had her, would we not have had her? Probably we wouldn't have. But I look at her and she is just such a wonderful gift, such a wonderful little child! I can't imagine not having her. But, maybe we would have adopted.

Five women underwent tubal ligations to assure they would not have more children. Three husbands of affected women had vasectomies, and three affected men also had vasectomies. These were all childless at the time of the procedure.

The seventeen never-married single subjects, some in their thirties or forties, had grown up with far more knowledge about their condition than the older subjects and were, in almost every instance, vehement about not having children. Women often cited the consideration of their condition becoming worsened, as well as the concern about passing on NF1. Said Angela:

Even now that I'm engaged, it's very hard. It takes all types, but not for me. It's a hard decision. And every time we make love, I do worry about getting pregnant. I do worry about it. Oh! I can't tell you. When we first became lovers, every time we made love, I'd go into the bathroom and give myself more injections of spermicide. I'm telling you, the money that I've spent for the Ortho company!

I think we are going to have to order out: I think we're going to have to adopt. You know, my health is at risk. I'm not willing to go through more trouble with this, or to have a child with NF. I mean I can't do it, as much as I would like to have children. I can't. I know how horrible it was to grow up with this.

And Terry:

These fifty-fifty odds are too high for me to take. I would never, ever have a child after the hell I have gone through growing up. The only women with NF that I have seen are the people on television shows, and these are very hard for me to watch. They have said their conditions really accelerated during pregnancy, and that is something I don't want to have happen.

Six single men had made the decision not to have children, and in most cases this was tantamount to their opting not to marry. For instance, said Hal:

Once I found out that there's a fifty-fifty chance of passing it on, it's kind of like, "Well, do I want to start a relationship that I know is doomed for failure anyway?"

Why do you think it would necessarily be that?

All the girls that I know want to have kids. I mean that's a priority. For me, it's kind of like, "Well, if you marry me, we aren't having kids." You can adopt them, but for them, it's kind of like, "Well, I want my own." So why set yourself up for that inevitable, dead-end relationship? Just say, "If a relationship comes along, fine. If it doesn't, I'm definitely missing out on a part of life, but I'm not depressed about it. It's just the way it is."

And Randy:

I get involved with women who tell me that they want kids; I tell them I don't. I can't be a father. I can adopt and I can raise a child, but I can't be a blood father. I think I'd be a good role model and a good father figure. I can be a daddy; I can't be a father. I think I'd make a great daddy, but being a father is someone who sires a child.

Follow-up interviews portrayed the ambivalence of a number of women about having children. Several who had been quite definite about not having children changed their minds over a three-year period. Said Cecilia early in our interviews:

Not only do I have to think of the child I'm going to be carrying, but I have to think about how it affects me. When and if I get pregnant, I'm going to have to worry about more tumors. It's something I can't reverse. And that scares me. So when I see people and they've got a cute little baby and I get jealous, I say, "Okay, Cecilia, the fact is, you have a genetic disease and they don't." The majority of people could probably have a normal kid and not pass anything on to it. But do people like me have the right to keep passing on genetic defects? I mean it's not really fair to the children.

But maybe I would be able to handle a child with it because I would give her love and talk to her about it, and let her know she's still okay. When I was growing up I felt ugly and deformed inside and I didn't have anybody telling me, "That's not true." So, I would definitely tell my daughter or son that she or he was lovable and pretty and still loved.

When my boyfriend and I talked about kids, I said, "Well, there's two things you should know—that I can pass it on," and that didn't seem to bother him. Then I told him about the increase of tumors. And I said I didn't know if I could handle having more tumors. He assured me that he would still love me. I said, "Yes, yes, but that's not the point." I said, "You're not with me twenty-four hours a day to have your arms around me and say, 'It's okay, I love you.' I have to deal with myself; I have to go to work; I have to be out there in the world and I don't know if I can handle having all those tumors." I told him I'd love to have children, but maybe we would have to talk about adoption or surrogate.

However, even in this period Cecilia was inconsistent in using birth control, and thought several times that she was pregnant because her monthly period was late. Three years later, and soon to be married, she was seriously considering having a baby.

Now we're thinking about having a baby. The geneticist told us we could test the fetus for NF but I don't think I want to. If we want a kid bad enough, I can't see getting pregnant and, let's just say two months is when they do the test, being pregnant for two months, being all excited about having a kid, having the test, the test says the baby has NF, and then having an abortion. And besides, even if the test is positive, they can't say how bad the NF would be. I don't think I'd want to know for nine months that I'm carrying a baby with NF. Because then, am I doing the right thing? Oh my God, is she going to be deformed? I think I'd rather not know. If we want a kid that badly, and we're willing to accept that it has NF, then we don't do the testing.

And then as for tumors, the doctor says, "You'll get a few more, but you're not going to get thousands." And I say, "Oh, okay, that's comforting to know, I'm not going to get thousands," and he says, "Maybe you won't get *any* more." But there are people that *have* gotten thousands. But my fiance says he can't understand why I am so concerned about tumors. He said, "Well, you've lived with this almost your whole life. Why haven't you gotten used to it? So we have a child that has some, and suppose you get some more tumors; I'll still love you." So he just doesn't think it's any big issue.

A similar case was Rosa whose thinking also shifted from the time I had initially interviewed her three years before when she was single.

My husband and I are thinking about, well, maybe having a baby. Even with the risk factors involved, I really want to have a child. I mean it's very strange for me to say this because the whole time when I was growing up I always said, "I'm never having children because of the fact that I have this disease." But never having children is a long time to say "never." I really never thought I would change my mind about having children, but I guess I was too young to make a decision like that at that age. I guess that is what it comes down to.

Norita went so far as to discuss reversing the tubal ligation she had had at twenty-two, but her physician said that her chances of conceiving were slim and Norita could not afford the reversal procedure.

The increased incidence of tumors during pregnancy is a definite possibility. Five subjects reported that their tumors noticeably increased during pregnancy. Grace commented to me that with each of her three pregnancies more tumors came. "They seemed to pop up overnight." Lou said that when she was pregnant with her son her tumors grew "like wildflowers. When I went to the doctor to have a few that were bothering me removed, first he put down 'One hundred tumors or more' and then he scratched out 'one hundred' and he put down 'thousands.' "

Adult children sometimes expressed their concerns about their birth having exacerbated their mother's condition. Victor has thought many times that if his mother had not borne him her NF1 might have been less severe. "I heard that she could hardly tell she had the disease until after she had me. Then the hormonal changes took effect and that is what caused the nodules to appear. Every time she had a kid they showed up more and more."

Huson (1994a:192) has pointed up the fact that studies have shown a reduction in relative fertility in affected persons in comparison with the general population. In keeping with the patterns of the subjects reported in this volume, Huson and others found that men with NF1 tend to marry less than women with NF1 and are less likely to have children. I found that even though women chance the exacerbation of their own condition in addition to the 50 percent possibility in each pregnancy of passing on the condition, they clearly are still more ready to have children than are men.

HARD DECISIONS

Comprehensive mapping of the human genome promises to yield detailed information for preconception and prenatal testing, allowing for greater choices and much more deliberate family planning than has been possible to this time. Preconception testing will inform prospective parents about the genetic characteristics they might pass on to their children. Postconception or prenatal testing can reveal numerous genetic conditions that may affect parents' choices of carrying a fetus to term or opting for abortion. (See Bobinski 1996 for a comprehensive discussion of genetic issues and reproductive decision-making.) Asch and Geller (1996) have noted that as prenatal screening becomes more precise, societal and political pressures may grow to persuade persons who are carriers of genetic disorders not to have children or to selectively abort.

Decisions based on information from prenatal testing in dominant conditions like NF1 constitute a sometimes unsettling intersection or even collision of ideological orientations from reproductive and disability rights perspectives and from a range of feminist points of view. The reproductive rights movement and feminist perspectives demand women's freedom to choose to carry or opt for abortion for any child for any reason. Prenatal testing allows a woman the opportunity to choose abortion for a particular fetus which may carry a disability "undesirable" to the parents. Medical ethicists and disability rights activists have shown concern about parents opting for abortion because of features some may consider less than serious or even frivolous.

A number of researchers and activists have pointed up the social implications of aborting a fetus because of genetic issues, stating that this choice represents a rejection of children with disabilities and a move to a society with less physical differentiation. Indeed, there are few positive role models in the United States for mothering a disabled child (Finger 1992). Asch and Geller in discussing this difficult and sensitive topic state:

we remain concerned that avoiding the problems that may come with diagnosable disability by using selective abortion may ultimately erode our tolerance of difference as a society, and our conceptions of ourselves as people who should adapt and master the many turns that life brings. We fear that ultimately, children will not be served well if their opportunity for joining the human family and community rests on their having some set of cognitive and physiological characteristics. (Asch and Geller 1996:339)

Rachel, a politically aware person, focused on this issue after telling me she could not bear to bring a child into the world who might have to experience the problems she has.

But there are some bad times for me, not wanting to have a child with NF. To be called "genetically defective," I mean, it's like Nazis. What I can say is, that the ethos of the concentration camps is here. In fact, I always feel schizophrenic because I'm a supporter of free choice and abortion and genetic counseling and amniocentesis and that women have a right to choose how they run their lives and run their bodies, but I always feel a little twinge when I realize that it's generally deformed babies that are being aborted. Most of my friends who have babies have healthy babies, but abort the deformed babies. I always gasp because *I* would have been aborted! And, *I* would abort if I had a genetically deformed child. It just makes me a little nervous because society needs to have all kinds of people in it.

In the case of NF1 in addition to the ideological issues that women might bring to their reproductive choices, several considerations peculiar to NF1 also enter into their decision making. It is highly probable that the visibility and sometimes severity of a woman's condition will be permanently increased by pregnancy, although the extent of this increase cannot be known in advance. Secondly, the severity of a child's condition or which of the multitude of possible symptoms of NF1 a child might have cannot be predicted from existing tests. The severity of the mother's condition is not a prediction of a child's condition. Thus, women with NF1 frequently have found themselves mired in a conundrum with no easy answers. At the time the persons in this study made their reproductive choices, there were few genetic counselors available to assist them in their dilemmas. Persons who face these issues today may benefit greatly by seeking referrals to these professionals who are expert in the complexities around reproductive decision making.

While many persons with NF1 make the decision not to have children on the basis of their own painful experiences with physical problems they do not wish to see their children deal with, no doubt many others make this decision based on their own poor self-image and feelings of devalued status. The frequent humiliations they experienced in school and work contexts may seriously color their expectations for a good life for any children they may have affected by NF1. In contrast, in recent years profoundly short persons in Little People of America have asserted their improved feelings of self-worth and expectations for a good life for their children in the rapidly growing birth rate of dwarf children. A total environment more hospitable for little people is more responsible for this change of heart than physical problems around dwarfism. This issue will be discussed further in the Conclusion.

9

*Gender Response**

During a discussion about men's and women's responses to NF1, Elise commented:

Being human beings, men and women are not that much different in our humanness. We want to be loved; we want to be accepted; we want to be attractive; we want to be able to perform in whatever it is. So I just can't believe that a man with NF would be less affected emotionally than a woman.

Twenty-eight persons, fourteen men and fourteen women, were queried specifically about gender response to NF1. While less than half of these twenty-eight adults had any knowledge of others with the condition through attending support groups or having affected family members, none were loathe to express themselves about gender response. Their opinions tended to be based on their own beliefs and experiences, and also on commonly held stereotypes about how men and women experience pain or appearance negatively valued in American society.

Subjects tended to comment on whether they thought NF1 was "harder" on men or women, and how men or women would cope with their condition. The responses were divided equally among the three alternatives of (1) there is no difference between men's and women's responses, (2) NF1 is harder on women, and (3) NF1 is harder on men. The responses of men and women were essentially also equally divided in each of these three groups. Typically those in the first category believe response depended on the person's attitude, not gender. For example, said Clarise:

*Portions of this chapter are reprinted from *Social Science and Medicine*, Vol. 42, No. 1, Joan Ablon, Gender Response to Neurofibromatosis 1, pp. 99–109, copyright 1996, with permission from Elsevier Science.

I don't think it matters whether you're a male or female. I think your personal attitude is what is going to make a difference. I think it is all in your head, I mean what kind of attitude you give yourself.

And Lily:

I think that we're a society that's so hung up on our bodies that men, if they have a lot of tumors on their torso, and certainly if they have them around the groin, or if they have them on their penis, would be concerned. Rebecca is very sensitive because she has so many on her breasts and her stomach. When she was dating she never wanted anybody to touch her because she knew that they would feel them through her clothing, and they would wonder what they were feeling. I can't imagine that a man wouldn't have the same thought if he had them on his torso. So I think there are concerns of how a member of the opposite sex, let alone your own sex, is going to view you if they see you naked with all these tumors. I think it would be just as difficult for a man as for a woman. I think how you react to it is largely based on how you're raised.

I think a woman may worry about the children more. I think that if you have NF and you're the one pregnant, that a woman might worry more about giving birth to a child with NF than a man who has NF. He's not the one who's pregnant. He's not the one looking at the changes in his body, or developing more tumors while he's pregnant.

I think a lot of it boils down to how severely you're affected with the NF. If you're affected severely I don't think it matters if you're a man or a woman, you're going to share common fears and feelings.

"WOMEN HAVE A HARDER TIME"

Most of those who felt that either men or women have a harder time were very emphatic about what they felt the differences to be. Slightly more women than men stated that they think women have a harder time. About half of this number stated that their beliefs were based on issues of appearance—that women in our society are judged more harshly on their appearance. Some brought up issues of child-birth—that women ultimately have to make the decisions about having children, even though an affected father can equally pass on the condition. Others stated that men look at the issue more dispassionately, and thus are less psychologically affected. Said Maureen:

Maybe it's going to be worse for me because I'm a woman and what you still see in all the TV is the body beautiful type, and having the beautiful complexion. For a man, they're supposed to be more rugged. And they always end up with shirts that are down to their wrists, where a woman will be more revealing, with the type of dresses you might wear in the summer time. You know how men are always looking at women and women are trying to make themselves nice looking. Women are more conscious of their appearance.

And Robert:

I think if you look at it from a point of view that a woman would like to feel that she looks nice. But me, I could care less. For instance, if my wife had the spots on her back that I have, she probably would not go to her swimming classes. If I wanted to go to exercise, I would go, because I don't care. It doesn't bother me, and I don't think it's going to bother other people either. You can transfer your psychology to someone else by making them feel that you're not bothered by it, and they shouldn't be that much either.

And Lou:

It's more okay for a man to have disfigurement. Look at the society we live in. If a woman is ten pounds overweight she's looked at as a freak.

And several other women thought men respond differently because culture dictates that men are supposed to be stronger, more "macho" and try to get on with their lives sooner.

Rachel pointed up the general differences between the way men and women are raised in this society:

Well, I think there's a difference just how men and women respond on anything, given our culture, given the socialization of baby boys and baby girls. Having never been a man, of course, I'm going to have to really just delve into stereotypes. I think that men probably respond with, "It's not that bad, I'm tougher; I'm going to hide my hurt and hide my injuries, my social wounds." So I think they'd probably come off as a little nonchalant. A little more *laissez faire* about things, which may or may not be true. I mean their real feelings, when given permission to have them and given a safe place to express vulnerability, would probably just be the same as anyone. But men are never given that permission.

"MEN HAVE A HARDER TIME"

For those who said men have a harder time with NF1, the reasons ranged from economic to psychological. Some specified the conditions for which NF1 could be harder for a male. The profound impact of appearance on the potential for a normal social and sexual life is apparent in the following responses. Susan noted:

Because NF makes it less possible to be physically active, you don't have the jock option, so men are probably more compromised than women because men are socially expected to be a jock, to be physically active. But I think their chances for dating and marriage are very minimal and slim. They're as compromised as a woman with NF. I'm sure a man's response about sexuality is the same as any woman, that when you have a nonstandard body you feel as if you're living a half life because you're not living a sexual life.

In keeping with Susan's comments, Reggie stated:

From a man's standpoint, anything that makes you feel less manly, like if you're disfigured in some way or if you're not attractive to women, the less normal you are, the more poor your self-image is—especially if you can't express your sexuality. If you sublimate all of your sexual energy because you don't think any woman would have an interest in you, and if she did, it would only be because of curiosity, you start carrying that around, and after a while it gets pretty heavy.

I think that the more disfigured or impacted people with NF are, whether it's by the tumors, or by whatever, wouldn't be that much different from someone who had another serious physical ailment. I don't know why it would be different for a man than a woman, but I think that it may be more a function of just how they perceive their disability and how they perceive themselves because of the disability, than it does with the disability itself. I think that there are some people who when life gives them a lemon, they make lemonade. And maybe a greater percentage of women than men do that and just kind of do the best they can with what they have.

Thoughtfully, Sarah, in her usual analytic manner, pointed up a variety of economic and social implications:

I think that a disfigured woman is far more devalued as a human being than a man is. I think it's harder on a woman. But, I also tend to think that, at least in our society, there is still enough sexism left that a disfigured man may be affected more in terms of his employability, because he's expected to support a family, probably more so than a woman. I also think that if a good-looking man *or* woman applied for a job and a disfigured person came in and applied for the same job, I'm sorry, they are going to take the good-looking person. I think that men have it harder if they are disfigured and for purposes of employability are devalued on the basis of disfigurement.

But women are devalued on both levels. It is more acceptable for a man to have a scar and so on. Women may be devalued by our whole culture because they are not beautiful *and* because they are disfigured. And then the double bind to that is that you're out in the community expecting to be hired. So I am full of contradictions because I can't figure out which one is harder. It is a little difficult to try and sort out which gender has more problems.

Four women commented that women confront and take hardship and illness better than men. For example, Isabelle:

I think women deal with just about anything that's bad in their lives better than men. Men like to be in control and don't like to have anything happen to them that they can't control. And women, I think, because they've had children and because women are such second-class citizens and treated as such, that they can cope better. I know when I was in rehab at both the University and City Hospitals, the women patients dealt a lot better with what was happening to them than the men patients. Men patients wouldn't accept it. They'd be in this wheelchair and they were told they would never walk again, and they still wouldn't accept it. They'd say, "I'll walk again; I'll walk again; I'm not going to stay in this goddamn wheelchair the rest of my life." Where a woman would say, "All right, tell me what I have to learn to do. What do I have to do to adjust to this?"

And Lou:

It matters how bad the person's NF is, and if it's a male or female. Probably because men's egos are so different. Men have weird, different kind of egos.

Weird?

You know, strange egos. They just think they're hot stuff. I think women can take pain more than men can anyway. So I think they could cope with it better than men can. Because, God, they get a little cold and they cry. They're really in bad shape, those guys. It's unreal.

SUPPORT GROUP MEETINGS

I asked subjects about the paucity of men at support group meetings. At most of the meetings I attended over a four-year period less than 20 percent of those present were males, and the few males in attendance tended to be nonaffected fathers of affected children, or occasionally, nonaffected spouses or partners of affected women.[1] I asked subjects why they thought there was this differential gender ratio. Men essentially stated unequivocally that men do not wish to face up to problems, and even if there are problems, they do not want to acknowledge them in public. The terms "macho" and "male ego" were used numerous times. For example, Edward:

I just suspect that support groups in general are much more popular with females than men, because it's a pure macho "I don't need support" attitude that a lot of men have. It's part of our basic socialization. I don't know whether you'd find that same characteristic in any support group, but it wouldn't surprise me. As for me, I don't think I have anything to give and I don't think I have anything to get. There are some people that love to go and parade their woes in public and unburden themselves to anyone who will listen. That's their own particular way of coping with whatever they have to cope with. Not mine.

Other men said they did not want to deal with personal feelings. Said Randy:

I know the reason I don't go is that I just don't want to have to deal with my personal feelings. I know that we, as men, are taught not to show our emotions. We're taught that we're not supposed to be close; we're not supposed to be emotional; we're not supposed to give of ourself.

And Rudy:

Men are used to doing things by themselves. They normally do not open up. If there is a problem men are more likely not going to admit it. They are so used to dealing with things one-to-one, while women share things. The relationships between women and girls, especially when growing up, are much closer than guys have. Women share these inner secrets whereas guys make jokes back and forth about what not. It is not a real sharing. Especially now, when women seem to be supporting each other more and men seem to be supporting each other less, this is why the divorce rate is so high.

Women's opinions were akin to those of men, citing cultural patterning as an inhibiting influence. Said Terry:

Well, it's like in Al-Anon meetings or in self-help meetings or in self-help classes or in any of those kinds of things, you see mostly women. And men in our culture are raised to ignore what they're feeling and what their symptoms are and everything involved with what they have. I kind of feel sorry for men in our culture because they're always like the Simon and Garfunkel song, "I am a rock; I am an island."

And Sharon:

Men don't share their feelings. It is okay for a woman to say, "I need help; I need support; I need to talk to other people about this and get that support." It is not okay for men. Macho men don't need groups like that; men don't cry; men don't have feelings and all that. I think that is a bunch of hooey and I think that is too bad because you could really get some good networking there if you have both men and women.

SOCIAL BEHAVIOR

The social lifestyles of many male subjects are very different from those of women. Of the thirty-two women, twenty, about two-thirds, are currently married; and five are divorced. Seven, or less than one-fourth, are never-married singles. Their profile differs markedly from that of the men. Of twenty-two men, ten, or under one-half, are married; two are divorced; and ten, or almost another half, are never-married singles. While these numbers are small, all subjects were recruited in the same manner and had comparable visibility and severity of their NF1 conditions.

The differences in lifestyles and attitudes toward social life and relationships are significant in seven of the ten single men from those of any of the single women. In fact, five single men, or about one-fourth of the total, appear to have retreated from social life very early on. Concomitantly with early learning disorders that were not aggressively dealt with in their school years twenty to thirty-five years ago, these men frequently have developed negative self-images and had poor educational histories. Physical symptoms of NF1 were moderately visible in the teen years of three of the five. Although physical symptoms are apparent now in their thirties and forties, these symptoms are not more severe than those of many of the women in the sample. The men hold jobs that would be considered more marginal than do the women—jobs with low incomes that may further decrease these men's value in their own eyes. Most of them have dated very little or not at all. The interviews reflect minimal sexual experience as compared to the single women in my sample, many of whom have had considerable sexual experience, no matter their degree of severity or how visible their appearance. In fact, my interviews with single or divorced women in every case dealt with their concerns about relationships and marriage. We often talked about strategies for meeting men!

The persistence of many women was illustrated by this statement of a woman in her forties who has made heroic efforts over the years to meet men:

You could always go your whole life saying "what if" or "if only." I've tried a dating service and also personal ads, and they haven't worked out, but I figure what do I have to lose if I don't try? I'll just be sitting home in my closet. I went out with some of these men and they were just so rude. They were awful. But I'll keep on trying!

The single men tended to be much more resolute about not having children than were the single women, most of whom were very ambivalent about this highly charged issue. Having made a pragmatic decision not to have children for fear of passing on their NF1, the men feel disqualified for marriage.

They all presented a number of reasons why they have not dated and do not expect to marry. Larry, a thirty-one-year-old man, apparently has been discouraged from dating because of the words of a schoolgirl who rejected him seventeen years ago!

I don't have any steady girlfriend, one that I go out with. I often wonder, if I didn't have these nodules on me, would that make me different somehow? Because I think that they must be thinking, "What's wrong with him, what does he have?"

Is there anyone you've asked out?

Yeah, there was this one gal I asked out. She said, "No one is going to get married to you."

How old was she?

We were both fourteen years old. That has always stuck in the back of my mind.

Said Rudy, a forty-year-old man:

Ordinarily I'm very aggressive, which I think comes from dealing with so many doctors and surgeons, but on a one-to-one level with young women I'm very shy. I still don't date, essentially. Psychologically, that's probably the hardest thing. Also I can't have kids.

And Jim, a forty-five-year-old man:

I don't earn enough to date. Right now, according to some of the guys I work with, they said dinner dating now is a hundred dollars. If you don't hit the liquor you could probably get it down to maybe about forty or fifty dollars, but when you get the liquor, by the time you get to adding it up, it's about a hundred. It's cheaper to go take my dog out to the burger stand, than to take a female out right now.

The five men who seem the most withdrawn from the prospect of getting married speak of themselves as "loners" from childhood, with most of the reasons springing directly or indirectly from their own or their parents' NF1. Several state that they enjoy children and have friends with small children. Thus they enjoy family life vicariously on the fringes of the lives of others.

Two women subjects repeatedly detailed the lives of affected young adult men in their families who also followed the pattern described above. Said Clarise about her affected brother:

Standing back and looking at my brother, I'd have to say that since the man is the one that has to ask for dates and pursue the woman, I'm sure my brother did not have very much self-confidence or self-esteem to ask a woman out. As far as we can tell, we don't think he had a first date until he was twenty-nine. And he ended up marrying her. And we're pretty sure my brother was a virgin when he married. My brother spent a lot of his time by himself in his room, doing his stamp collection or coin collection, or he was a cub leader. That's what he did on Friday nights. Occasionally he went camping with the boys. But we never heard him call any girls; we never saw him bring any over.

In my process of trying to understand the pattern of men who seemingly withdraw from social situations where women with comparable clinical conditions do not, I spoke with a number of thoughtful subjects about this. Rachel, one of the most analytic, came forward with these statements:

I'm not surprised about the men. The women are still somehow or another programmed to fantasize about getting married and having children, and they're out there trying, but I think it's all fantasy. Because we're as equally compromised as men and we're in the same boat. It is that we've just been socialized differently. Women are given permission to fantasize.

But women keep trying, even with tumors. For most of the men I know, their damage seems to have come from learning disabilities. They don't have as many tumors as the women, so the fact is, they could carry off "a one night stand" like some women do, but they don't. Why don't they?

Bad social cues. They've also been compromised socially. Learning disabilities have two concentrations. One, the actual pathology of not being able to process learning in the same easy manner that some children can, and also the pathology has a social impact; it has a school impact.

When you say the cues, what kind of cues do you mean?

Cues that started when they were wee ones.

So that they feel like on some level no one would want them?

How would anyone want them on *any* level? By the time you get to be an adolescent when you're incredibly vulnerable to begin with, even without NF, and never get a chance to graduate emotionally, you're still very emotionally immature.

So that particular emotional immaturity makes you feel you're out of the game then? And you just stay out of the game and you psyche yourself so that it doesn't hurt to be out of the game?

Absolutely.

You're not talking about social cues for the immediate moment, such as if they were to go to a bar and not "pick up" on somebody?

Right. Because you don't even opt into the system. You're totally removed, and you set things up to stop the pain from being so acute, that you're not even bothering with the pain, it doesn't exist. They're just "lumps and bumps." This is all subconscious. But I just see that women have more permission to fantasize. It's set up for us to fantasize.

So "Hope springs eternal in the human breast . . . "

Sure, as long as it's the female breast, as long as it's got boobs.

MALE STOICISM

A strong consensus was apparent in both men's and women's opinions about men's stoicism and reticence in help-seeking. My interviews with male subjects clearly demonstrated that in most cases stoicism and reticence indeed was the situation. While individuals of both sexes were gravely concerned about their health and appearance, men's concerns were couched in a much more matter-of-fact, practical, and detached manner. In American society men typically do not have the cultural permission to be emotional, admit personal disaster, or seek support. The following men's statements illustrated the practical approach to their condition exhibited by many men. Not one woman expressed her concerns in this manner. Said Michael:

I rarely go to doctors. Well, why bother? You can't do anything about it. Moaning, groaning, crying about it won't do any good. I can't say, "Kaazam" and snap my fingers and, "poof," it will go away. So, I've got to live with it. I'm thirty-five years old and it has not really slowed me down yet. I could live another thirty-five years and by that time I will be seventy and at that age, well, who cares?

And Hal, who had had a recent limb amputation for a malignant tumor:

I don't think about it. It's just a part of me. I would like to know what the future holds, but on the other hand, I can't, so I just live life day to day and take life as it comes. I don't have to worry about it. I'll just let it go and let life take its course as long as I can function reasonably well and as long as it doesn't slow me down.

And Benjamin:

I don't worry about it. If I die from it, I die from it. If it kills me, it kills me. We're all going to die. How we're going to die, we don't know. But if it kills me, it better help somebody else out, because if it didn't, I'm going to feel pretty bad.

Benjamin did die from NF1-related problems during the course of this research.

DISCUSSION

The literature on gender and disability reports that women with disabilities fare worse than men in economic and social life experiences. Disabled women tend to have less education than do men, to be unemployed more and receive less rehabilitation training. When working, they tend to be in lower-wage jobs and have lower levels of disability coverage and insurance benefits. They are more likely to live in families with incomes at or below the poverty level. Further, women's attractiveness is more significant for educational, work, and social opportunities. Women with disabilities are less likely to be married, and if they are, they are more likely to divorce. Disabled men often cope through the efforts of their wives. Disabled women are more likely to identify themselves as "disabled" than are men (Fine and Asch, 1985, 1988). Hanna and Rogovsky (1993) note, "there are special consequences of the intersection of being female and disabled" (p. 109). In keeping with these findings, Sitlington et al. (1992) report that women with mild disabilities after a year out of high school were found to have adjusted less well to adult life than did men. They had greater unemployment, and when employed, they held less desirable jobs, made less money, and received less benefits.

Varied types of disabilities may exact their particular price in relation to gender. The disabilities incurred in NF1 typically entail learning disabilities that may involve special considerations not often surveyed for their salience in the general literature, and an appearance that may be "unsightly" as judged by American cosmetic prescriptions. However, visible physical symptoms appear not to have held back many of the women subjects, except in very extreme cases. Learning disabilities appear to have hindered many men more in job aspirations and opportunities, and their inability to earn good wages contributed to their shying away from dating and the economic responsibilities of marriage. Further, early forceful decisions not to have children seemed to preclude marriage for many men. Indeed, a large proportion of the men in this study well illustrate the pattern of isolation that Hanna and Rogovsky (1993) report for women: "Most women with disabilities are clearly not full or equitable participants in American society" (p. 110).

Early learning disabilities that appear to have made both boys and girls vulnerable at home and at school may have more crucially affected male children. It may be that these early learning disabilities and related problems that created tentative and poorly performing children in the household of orientation and in school academic and sports activities, the chief arenas where the child's self-image is developed, precluded the development of assertiveness, independence, and proactivity. In accordance with societal expectations, male children are typically expected to be forceful and aggressive in their interactions with the world. Poor school achievement often resulted in negative self-images and ill-paying and low-status jobs. For some men the conviction that they should not pass on their condition resulted in an expectation of childlessness almost of the character of infertility. Nachtigall et al. (1992:119) have demonstrated that men with male factor infertility experience stigma because of inability to impregnate. "Their gender identity is affected by their failure to meet gender role expectations. Moreover, men commonly confuse potency with virility, and therefore men's sexual adequacy is threatened by a male infertility factor." Thus by the young adult years, some men affected by NF1 could be self-defined as quadruple failures in appearance, educational performance, economic achievement, and reproductive ability.

In contrast to the disparities in various consequences of disability that other researchers have reported to exist for men and women, my data suggest that a substantial percentage of the men in this study, although to all appearances able-bodied, do not have a "relatively positive" self-image, that they do identify as "disabled," or at least "imperfect," and have lower rates of marriage, and also proportionately poorer economic achievement than do women with comparable conditions. The multifaceted symptoms of NF1 appear to have caused them to perceive themselves as locked out of many normative arenas of life. Why five male subjects out of a total of twenty-two were thrust early into a pathway of social withdrawal while others who appear to have been affected by similar levels of NF1 symptoms did not, remains unclear. However, it is clear that not one female in this sample reacted in this manner, no matter the nature of her appearance, NF1 severity, or learning disorders. Many of these men were clearly seriously maimed because of early messages of their general undesirability.

Gilligan has described differences between men and women in their "models for a healthy life cycle." She states that men are more "distant" in their relationships. Gilligan generalizes that close friendships with a man or a woman are rarely experienced by American men. In contrast, "identity for women is defined in a context of relationship and judged by a standard of responsibility and care" (1982:160). "Women's sense of integrity appears to be entwined with an ethic of care, so that to see themselves as women is to see themselves in a relationship of connection" (1982:171). For men, "instead of attachment, individual achievement rivets the male imagination, and great ideas or distinctive activity defines the standard of self assessment and success" (1982:163). Following Gilligan's argument, some men with NF1 who are confronted by early failure realize on some level that there will be no "great ideas or distinctive activity" in their lives. For them perhaps the failure or inability to meet these criteria for manhood in our society makes even more improbable the lesser goal of establishing intimate relationships.

Although NF1 may have significant impact on both men and women in diverse and crucial areas of life, men may be more strongly affected psychologically, socially, and economically, despite their seemingly matter-of-fact pragmatic public style of acceptance. Their NF1 condition appears to have struck more centrally to the core of their manhood and personhood, disenfranchising them from many of the life-cycle accomplishments that help normalize individuals in our society.

NOTE

1. When I discovered that I was recruiting considerably fewer men than women for this study because fewer men attended NF support group meetings, I placed a notice in a support group mailer stating that I particularly wished to speak with men. Six men immediately responded by mail or telephone saying they would be happy to talk with me but did not wish to go to a support group meeting. Further, I was surprised to notice that five of the first six men I interviewed had spinal tumors, a symptom that could pose potentially serious problems, while none of the fifteen or more women I had interviewed to that time had spinal tumors. Because most symptoms of NF1 are thought to occur equally across the sexes, I propose the explanation that many men would have to be threatened by the loss of mobility or life before they would seek help or desire to talk to anyone at all about their condition.

10

Living with Uncertainty

Norita spoke with me about her many problems in growing up with NF1. It was clear that the many uncertainties around her condition were daily companions of her life:

All through my teens from the time I was thirteen till I was twenty I thought I was going to eventually look just like The Elephant Man. I believed that I was going to be "The Elephant Lady." That was why I didn't want to make any plans for the future, thinking, "What if I end up like that?" Now I really feel cheated because I know it was all a big mistake. It's no one's fault. I'm not blaming anyone. But that still is the stereotype now in people's minds.

Pam focused on the clinical uncertainties as well as those of appearance:

Whenever I have a new ache or pain that lasts for more than a week I think about it, "What is growing now?" Every once in awhile I get this really icky feeling, "What could be growing? Where could it be growing that I won't know about till it's too bad to be taken care of?"

Do you think it likely that it could be too bad to be taken care of?

No, but that is the rational side. I have two very distinct "me's," the rational and irrational.

I see the unpredictability of NF1 as its the most damaging psychological feature. Early dramatic statements of doctors and the media creation of The Elephant Man have provided the worst-case scenario for many of those affected, no matter how remote, or even impossible, the imagined symptoms might be. Even though it is now thought that The Elephant Man did not have NF1, the possibility of that vivid media-created image or another worst-case scenario still relentlessly dogs the footsteps of many affected persons and their families. Individuals and families manage *what could be* rather than *what is*.

For example to my question, "What do you think is the most worrisome aspect of NF1?" Pam brought up what she considered to be both her "rational" and "irrational" fears.

The most irrational worry, and I recognize that it *is* irrational, is that I'm going to look like The Elephant Man. I think the more rational fear is that I'm going to grow so many more of these neurofibromas and they might become malignant, that I'll die as a result. Perhaps that's also an irrational fear, but no knowledgeable medical person has ever been able to tell me whether or not that could happen. After all, the neurofibromas really started to grow steadily when I was thirty-four. They continue and I'm forty-two. They began to grow more on the body than the face, and I said, "thank God, I don't have any on the face." By the time I was thirty-eight or thirty-nine, they were really starting to grow on the face. One doctor told me that any kind of reconstructive or plastic surgery is impossible because, he said, "We'd have to cut away practically all of you that there is."

Did you read about The Elephant Man being rediagnosed? Did that make you feel any better about these possibilities?

No. The remote possibility may exist. It's just a big question mark.

When subjects were asked what they felt to be the most worrisome feature of NF1, most brought up some aspects of the uncertainty surrounding the condition. But even before this question, many discussed the uncertainty of NF1 and their fear of developing an unsightly appearance, becoming seriously ill or immobilized, or of a future experiencing a worsening of their ongoing specific health problems. Both men and women equally expressed this range of concerns.

DISFIGUREMENT

For most persons fears and anxieties related to disfigurement were the primary concern despite what other issues of greater clinical severity existed. It is a significant commentary on the specter of social stigma in subjects' lives that by far the fears and anxieties they expressed most frequently related to disfigurement. In contrast, the concerns of clinicians and their ranking of the severity of patients invariably is based on the seriousness of what are the least common problems of NF1 such as internal tumors or plexiform neurofibromas, loss of sight related to optic gliomas, or skeletal problems that could compromise mobility. However, the import of these was not primary for most persons. Said Harry, who had numerous internal tumors and lived in constant pain:

Rejection. I would say being rejected is the worst. The social aspect, as far as going out in the public eye, not just going for a job and getting rejected. The thing about The Elephant Man, and even though we know now that he didn't have NF, it's like people who have NF are still like that when they go outside, knowing that that kind of deformity is repulsive. Even though we have supposedly modernized, that we have come up the ladder, any kind of deformity is still repulsive and cannot be accepted yet.

And Jody:

I suppose the thing that may concern me is eventually growing facial tumors cosmetically more disfiguring than it is now, and that maybe I would eventually no longer be able to work, to teach. I hope and pray I'll never get like that. Dan has told me, "If that should happen in your case, I wouldn't love you any less. You would still be my wife, and I would still support you." Knowing that is important to me, that he's not going to reject me because I am no longer physically appealing. It's easy to say this now, because I don't have them in places where most people would see them.

Many persons talked about a fantasy of waking up one morning and finding that tumors have appeared on their face overnight, despite the fact that such a sudden explosion of tumors would be impossible. Said Rachel:

I don't have any tumors on my face now, but that doesn't mean that I won't always. And I live in terror that I'll wake up one morning, look in the mirror, and there they'll be. It is a very horrendous, terrifying nightmare I live. I always look. I mean, when I get up in the morning I close my eyes and I tap my face to make sure they haven't popped up during the night.

And Lacy:

Well, it's like a teenager having a pimple. He's going to wake up and there is going to be this huge pimple on his face. One of these days I am going to wake up and there is going to be one of them on the tip of my nose. Same with these tumors. I don't know when these things are going to pop up and be there. I used to count them. But it got to where I can't.

Several persons mentioned appearance as a concern but quickly added their fear that NF could kill them. For example:

I don't know how many I have but I can see more and more growing and I can see the tiny little bumps, the tiny little fibromas coming out and then I start thinking, "Oh, my God, I am going to get more and more five years from now." But what worries me the most is that I have one on my head and I am getting a lot of headaches lately. I wonder if this one is going to kill me.

SEVERE MEDICAL PROBLEMS

Next to disfigurement were fears about developing severe problems that could threaten life or mobility. Said Sharon:

The biggest worry is not knowing the final chapters. Thinking, "Oh, no, is that another tumor on the spine?" I try not to dwell on it. It's just the unknown. No one can say, "Okay, you're not going to have any more problems," or that, "These are the only problems you are going to have."

Nathan, who had had a recent operation for a malignant spinal tumor said:

I wouldn't wish this on anyone, even my worst enemy. It's with me all the time. And it's just sort of like a time bomb inside you ticking away. It could explode at any moment. Or it could *never* explode. It could be a big explosion; it could be a small explosion. It's just not knowing what's going to happen! I can't put aside a little ache or a pain. Every one is a serious issue until I do something. Usually it's nothing, but I have to go through the process of doctors, the tests, and waiting for the results. Is this going to be it? Is something going to happen?

Like I'm going through that now with this ringing in my ears. Is it the ears? Is it something in my brain? What is it? It may be something totally unconnected with NF, but the NF is just such a powerful force that it's the first thing I think of. I have very little control over it. I can have responsibility for it and try to do something about it when there's a problem by going to the right doctors and insisting on things. But there's really no control. It's being very much alone.

Nathan died of an undiagnosed massive brain tumor two months after our interview. And Lou:

The most dangerous thing is that you don't know where those little things are going to pop up. They may pop up in a vital organ. That is the most worrisome thing. They could pop up in your heart. In your brain. You don't know where. There is no warning. They just come. Then, sometimes they can be cancerous and sometimes they may not.

As Rachel told me:

For me, and I think true of most people—I worry where is it going to hit next? What will be some of the issues that I'm going to face? The hideous aspect of NF is that just because you don't have it doesn't mean you're not going to get it. The disease is progressive. Just because your kidneys aren't affected now, doesn't mean they're not going to be next week. So, what are the signs? What are the signs of aging and NF? What can I expect as a woman and have NF?

Several persons expressed their concern that their condition might become so severe that they would be unable to take care of themselves. Ronald, who had serious leg and back problems, told me soberly:

What worries me the most is that I'd have to totally depend on somebody else. That's scary! I'm not suicidal now, but it's still an option if the bottom line was "incapacitated." If total dependency was there, I'd certainly consider it. It absolutely terrifies me! If I just couldn't do for myself, and I couldn't be my own person. Nothing scares me more. If I found myself at the point where I'd be sitting there with tubes in me, and not be able to get up, not be able to go to the bathroom, life would lose its novelty. If I stay this way, it's not ideal, but it's okay. It's better than the alternative.

And Robbie:

I'm limited in my hearing. I don't know how far that's going to go, whether it's going to remain stable or I'm going to have my hearing diminished. I'm learning sign. I'm not being fatalistic thinking I'm going to go totally stone deaf. But it's more a matter that I'm preparing for the worst and expecting the best. So I want to learn as much as I can so that if it does happen, I'm going to be ready for it, and don't have to face a double trauma and have to learn a whole new language at the same time. I am having to make adjustments now for my hearing. I have to ask people to repeat themselves because I can't hear them.

Those persons who also had affected children invariably were more concerned about the possibility of serious problems for their children than for themselves. Two women who were in the throes of deciding whether to have children stated that the uncertainties around children were their main concerns.

ABSENCE OF ROLE MODELS

The anxiety created by the knowledge of a seemingly limitless variety of problems that could arise is not able to be mitigated by any realistic perceptions of role models. For example, in my prior research with unaffected parents of dwarf children, although they experienced the same emotions such as guilt, anger, or sorrow as have been reported for parents of other types of physically different children, when they could view and become acquainted with dwarf adults in the organization of Little People of America and saw that these were attractive and productive persons with jobs, homes, and families, their own children could become *normalized* in their eyes. Once they could absorb this concept of their child's dwarfism, they could start on a path of positive acceptance (Ablon, 1984, 1988). However, the parameters of achondroplasia and other most common types of dwarfism are fairly constant. Parents knew what they could expect in their child's development. With NF1 there seem to be *no* parameters. Likewise there are no widely known role models but The Elephant Man or the severely affected (but atypical) persons that have appeared on television programs. Most first-generation affected individuals I interviewed who did not attend support group meetings had never seen another person with NF1, or if they had, that person was often very visibly and/or severely affected.

Many persons dread going to support group meetings because they might see persons with multiple tumors or severe skeletal deformities. Norita told me she resisted going to meetings because she feared she might enter a room full of Elephant People. While some of the chief dynamics operative in most support or self-help groups are peer sharing, education, and role modeling, it appears that for many affected persons or parents of a child with NF1, the sharing of experiences and/or education and viewing of models do not necessarily provide confidence and freedom from fear, but to the contrary, may serve to provide a showcase for a multitude of symptoms and thus lead to the generation of even more anxiety. For example, Diane related her experience at the first support group meeting she attended.

> I went to this one meeting, my first one, and I cried all the way home, and then I cried some more at home. I was very taken aback. I wasn't sure I ever wanted to go to another meeting. There were people who were not as deformed as I was and there were people there who were more deformed. There was one woman who was my age, or maybe a little older, who had numerous tumors on her face. She came up to talk to me and said how beautiful I was. I thought, "I could look like that in ten years." It was very frightening to me to see that. Since my NF was not as pronounced as hers, she thought I was gorgeous. That was really scary.
>
> It is a very terrifying experience to see other people and wonder if that is going to happen to you. Especially if the people are older and you can see yourself in later periods of your life. You start to speculate, "When I am that age, or when I am sixty am I going to look this or that?" Or, "Is my five-year-old daughter going to look like that?"

Because there are few reassurances that professionals or other affected persons or their families can provide to counter or assuage their fears, many persons with NF1 live with anxiety about their condition as a chronic life companion.

11

The Specter of "The Elephant Man"[*]

The statements of two prominent geneticists characterize the major issues around the misdiagnosis of NF1 as The Elephant Man's Disease.

This is a classic case of good news and bad news. The good was that The Elephant Man association finally gave physicians and the public the idea that there was a disease out there called neurofibromatosis which most of them had never considered. The bad news is very obvious in that many families with NF who heard this association became frightened, particularly younger individuals who feared they would end up looking like The Elephant Man. (Francis Collins, Clinical geneticist and co-discoverer of the gene for neurofibromatosis 1, 1991)

Truly, such wide interest [in the Elephant Man] is a sociological phenomenon that can only be called elephant fever (EF). Experts in NF have not yet seen—nor are they waiting to see—a patient affected with "Elephant Man disease." . . . [T]he use of the term "Elephant Man" or "Elephant Man disease" is inhumane. Let's stem elephant fever and discourage the use of such terms. Let's take the EF out of NF. (M. Michael Cohen, Jr., Clinical geneticist and co-rediagnoser of "The Elephant Man's Disease," 1988)

The Elephant Man's Disease, the unfortunate misdesignation for NF1, a publicly little known or understood condition, acquired enormous notoriety through the portrayal of the life of Joseph Merrick, "The Elephant Man," on American stage, screen, and television. These portrayals, primarily in the 1970s and 1980s, parleyed

---

[*]Portions of this chapter are reprinted from *Social Science and Medicine*, Vol. 40, No. 11, Joan Ablon, "The Elephant Man" as "Self" and "Other": The Psycho-social Costs of a Misdiagnosis, pp. 1481–1189, copyright 1995, with permission from Elsevier Science.

this designation of Merrick's condition into a household phrase, a metaphor for the grimmest extreme of ugliness.

THE ELEPHANT MAN

Ashley Montagu's remarkable book, *The Elephant Man: A Study in Human Dignity*, first published in 1971, reprinted Sir Frederick Treves' vivid and moving twenty-five page account of John (better known as Joseph) Merrick from Treves' volume, *The Elephant Man and Other Reminiscences*, published in 1923. Treves, an internationally prominent British physician, encountered Merrick, who was living as a carnival attraction, and brought him to London Hospital where he lived in a sheltered and comfortable state for the next four years until his death at age twenty-five. Merrick became a *cause celebre* of his day and many prominent persons visited him in his hospital quarters. Treves described his first encounter with Merrick:

The showman—speaking as if to a dog—called out harshly: "Stand up!" The thing arose slowly and let the blanket that covered its head and back fall to the ground. There stood revealed the most disgusting specimen of humanity that I have ever seen. In the course of my profession I had come upon lamentable deformities of the face due to injury or disease, as well as mutilations and contortions of the body depending upon like causes; but at no time had I met with such a degraded or perverted version of a human being as this lone figure displayed. (Montagu 1971:15)

I supposed that Merrick was imbecile and had been imbecile from birth. . . . The conviction was no doubt encouraged by the hope that his intellect was the blank I imagined it to be. That he could appreciate his position was unthinkable. Here was a man in the heyday of youth who was so vilely deformed that everyone he met confronted him with a look of horror and disgust. He was taken about the country to be exhibited as a monstrosity and an object of loathing. It was not until I came to know that Merrick was highly intelligent, that he possessed an acute sensibility and—worse than all—a romantic imagination that I realized the overwhelming tragedy of his life. (Montagu 1971:18)

Treves closed his essay by saying:

As a specimen of humanity, Merrick was ignoble and repulsive; but the spirit of Merrick, if it could be seen in the form of the living, would assume the figure of an upstanding and heroic man, smooth browed and clean of limb, and with eyes that flashed undaunted courage.

His tortured journey had come to an end. All the way he, like another, had on his back a burden almost too grievous to bear. (Montagu 1979:37–38)

In his book Montagu speculated on the personality development of an individual so physically marked, and he presented a discussion of neurofibromatosis and genetic disorders. Montagu's resurrection of Treves' essay was the impetus for various plays that first depicted Merrick's story to society at large. Said Montagu in the preface to the 1979 edition of his book:

The response to the [1971] book has been quite astonishing. To my knowledge there exist at least half-a-dozen moviescripts and at least eight plays by different authors. Seven of these plays have been produced. As a report in *Variety* (7 March 1979) put it, "A herd of 'Elephant Men' is proliferating on U.S. stages." (Montagu 1979:xiv)

The poignant story of Merrick was subsequently popularized on stage, screen, and in print. For analyses of the similarities and differences in these accounts see Graham and Oehlschlaeger (1992). Books have included vivid photographs of Merrick alive, of postmortem casts, and of his skeleton (Montagu 1971, 1979; Howell and Ford 1980; Drimmer 1985).

While Treves labeled Merrick "A Case of Congenital Deformity" in an 1885 paper, dermatologists Crocker in 1905 and Weber in 1909 suggested that Merrick had neurofibromatosis. In 1982 the suggestion was challenged by several clinicians who examined his skeleton and they suggested that he had three diseases. In 1986 two Canadian geneticists called his condition "Proteus Syndrome" (Tibbles and Cohen 1986; Cohen 1988). While there is no consensus on the identity of Merrick's condition, it is now generally thought that it was not NF1.

In theatrical productions of "The Elephant Man" the title role was played without makeup leaving to the imagination the horror of his appearance. Most American viewers saw the moving picture or television film production in which Merrick was portrayed in graphic detail or accompanied by photographs taken during his lifetime that illustrated his physical characteristics.

The personal features of The Elephant Man were presented as tragically negative because of his inability to measure up to many important values of American audiences. These values tend to emphasize physical beauty, good health, economic success, and financial independence. Merrick was grossly deformed, unemployable, indigent, passive, and essentially totally dependent on others for his survival. He was, however, portrayed as a dignified and "sweet" person. Nonetheless, these positive personality features scantly balanced out all of the negatives in their lasting impression on public viewers.

I investigated both the consequences of the diagnosis of NF1 as The Elephant Man's Disease for those persons with the condition, and also the role of the diagnosis in the scientific quest to understand and find a cure for NF1. The enormous publicity generated by the books, plays, moving picture, and television film was significant for its effect on case finding for treatment and research. For example, American Medical News on February 20, 1981 stated, " 'Elephant Man' has its share of fear arousal, but it also has boosted physicians' efforts to understand a mysterious disease and brought hundreds of cases to light. . . . Clinics have been swamped with referrals from physicians and by inquiries from people who heard about the clinics on their own."

Chapters of the National Neurofibromatosis Foundation, Inc. utilized this publicity for fundraising around the country. Philip Anglim, an early leading actor of the off-Broadway production, appeared before Congress requesting more governmental funding for research. Further, some clinicians believe that the dramatic image of The Elephant Man also moved a number of scientists to join in the major effort of the past decade that resulted in the exciting discovery of the gene that causes NF1 in July 1990. One geneticist commented that prior to 1984 few scientists were interested in NF1. However, the grisly image of The Elephant Man provided a gestalt, a single but horrific example of a person with many serious complications of NF1. Because the condition has such an enormous variability of symptoms, it could be perceived as "just" a bunch of skin tumors and cafe-au-lait spots, the most common (and least severe) symptoms of NF1. Thus, NF1 did not appear to many scientists to have that much severity to study. In contrast to this perception, the dramatic case of The Elephant Man created a strong impression of a serious condition to which a scientist could valuably contribute. Reported this geneticist, a scientist might say, "Ah, now I have some context for NF1. This is a potentially serious condition, therefore it's worth my studying it. If I figure this out, it is really going to help people" (Carey 1990b).

By the mid-1980s NF1 was a condition "whose time had come." The complexity of the condition became attractive rather than daunting. The new technologies that were available could enable scientists to locate the chromosome on which the gene was based. Scientists could get caught up in the actual glory and fame of being the one that was recognized for mapping the gene.

In addition to querying subjects about The Elephant Man phenomenon, I also spoke with ten health professionals across the country—physicians and genetic counselors who see many NF1 patients in their practices, and with Ashley Montagu, whose book precipitated the media phenomenon of The Elephant Man. Affected individuals were asked a number of questions about their own and their family's responses to the books, plays, and films about The Elephant Man, and their attitudes toward using the label of The Elephant Man's Disease for NF1.

IMPACT ON AFFECTED PERSONS

What effect has the phenomenon of The Elephant Man had on those affected with the disorder? The clinicians that I spoke with felt that the dramatic image of The Elephant Man badly scared people with NF1. A neurologist who sees many patients with NF1 stated, "It scared the hell out of patients, particularly parents who would go crazy thinking that their child would grow into this monstrosity." Said one genetic counselor, "I think The Elephant Man is the biggest disservice ever done to people with NF1. Everyone comes wondering if they will look like that." Within the context of the unpredictability of the condition, early dire statements of doctors in combination with the media depiction of The Elephant Man greatly contributed to the burgeoning of subjects' fears.

During the 1980s doctors often associated NF1 with The Elephant Man's Disease when they talked with patients or parents about their own or their child's condition. One NF specialist commented that he found that the less knowledgeable doctors were about the condition, the more they were likely to use the term "The Elephant Man's Disease." Specialists typically explained to their patients that Joseph Merrick was a very extreme and atypical case. Now they must reassure patients that Merrick did not have NF1 at all.

A geneticist who sees many NF1 patients in his practice stated:

I know I evolved in the way I dealt with The Elephant Man in my counseling. I really was never convinced. Because I always had this concern that Merrick was the symbol of disfigurement and his case overstated the severity, I always felt the importance in pointing out to families that even if Merrick had NF1, his complications were rare. But I wasn't really convinced that he had it.

The greatest traumas occurred when the labeling was associated with the first diagnosis. In some cases friends and relatives rather than doctors made the first association for patients or their families. Said one mother:

When the doctor told me that Karen had The Elephant Man's Disease I fainted dead away on his floor. Then when I told my husband later that day I fainted again.

And another mother:

I went right to the medical libraries at the university and at Harper Hospital.

What was your reaction?

Horror, horror.

In the course of my interviewing I asked subjects a number of questions about the media representations of The Elephant Man. I asked if they had read the book or had seen one of the plays or films, their reactions in relation to their own or their child's condition, and whether they thought the media phenomenon was good or bad. I also asked them if they use the term "The Elephant Man" to explain their condition to others. Most had either seen the play or a film, or read the book.

Just over half of the affected adults questioned stated that they had experienced varying levels of depression, anxiety and/or fear at the association of their condition with the image of The Elephant Man. Said Cecilia:

I cried. I identified with him.

Were you crying for him or for yourself?

Probably for myself. But no, for him too, because I don't have to hide behind a mask like he did. And I also felt mad at the world because the world puts so much emphasis on beauty and perfection, you know, normality. And then when there's somebody that has something that's not normal you stare and don't accept them and make fun of them.

And Angela:

It was bad. First of all, I saw the play. I was hysterical because it was tapping into the awfulness of what my body looks like. And you saw the actor standing up straight and tall and then he gets the scoliosis and he cramps his body into that disgusting look. And then there was the description about the flabby skin and the smell. I had that. That's what my hips looked like before these surgeries. And I don't want to be associated with that. That's not what I have!

Slightly less than half of those questioned stated they felt that the case of The Elephant Man was so extreme that it was too remote from their condition to frighten them. For example, Mae said, "My sister who also has NF and I went to see the movie. We just never did relate any of that to us. He was just too badly effected. It didn't seem like anything our family had." And Loreen likewise felt, "There is no way that that is NF. It wasn't that I was denying it, but it would be like saying, 'Every Black person has sickle cell anemia.' I mean, no way. He was just too deformed."

Five persons stated that they refused to see the film or read the book. In some cases this was related to the specific stage they were in in their acceptance of their condition. For example said Luis:

When "The Elephant Man" first came out I didn't want anything to do with it. I was just tending to hide out. I was like a hermit. After I started going to more seminars [support group meetings] and talking to more people—it was like therapy. Then I decided to watch "The Elephant Man." I thought before that I was going to be deformed, but after I found out that I didn't have it as bad, that's when I decided to watch it.

Reggie said:

I'm glad the movie was made, but I don't want to see it. I read the book. I tried rereading it again recently and I read the first page and I had to put it down.

And Lou told me this story:

When I was in the hospital this doctor came in that was one of those doctors that you only see once, and he said, "Did you ever see that movie, 'The Elephant Man'?" I said, "No." Then he said, "Well, I think you should with your condition." He kind of snickered and the way he said it made me feel really icky, like he was making fun of me. I actually told him to get the hell out of my room. I didn't ever want to see "The Elephant Man" after that.

The great majority of the parents interviewed expressed horror at their child's association with the image of The Elephant Man. Those parents who did not have NF1 themselves had never seen another person with NF1, and thus had no role models to mediate the probability of their child looking like The Elephant Man. This was a significant contrast to the number of affected adults who felt that the association was clearly too remote from their own condition to be so frightening. Jim told me matter-of-factly, "My mother didn't want me to see that movie, but when she passed away five years ago, I went and watched it. My mother probably thought that I would get scared and go commit suicide if I watched that movie. But it didn't bother me."

ATTENTION BROUGHT BY THE PORTRAYAL

With only a few exceptions, all persons interviewed thought the attention brought by The Elephant Man to NF1 or to any severely different physical condition was a good thing, even though a number of these same persons had reacted badly to the portrayal themselves. Said Robbie, "I think it's nice. It focused on the disease. It's the same thing as when Rock Hudson declared he had AIDS. All of a sudden—gee, Rock Hudson! And people started getting interested, and I think it generated support for those people and may have generated some donations."

Most subjects stated that they explained their condition to other people by telling them that they have a mild form of The Elephant Man's Disease since "everyone" has heard of that. Those who knew about the rediagnosis tended to continue using the association, modifying their explanation to say that NF1 *used to be* thought of as The Elephant Man's Disease. Said Marilee:

I've only used it since I have been trying to explain to people in the community what our support group is about. For example, for a benefit event, I will explain that we are a group that is part of the National Neurofibromatosis Foundation. When people say, "The what?" I explain that they may not have heard of this condition but may have heard of it referred to as "The Elephant Man's Disease." Then they say, "Oh, yeah." Now, I hate doing this, but it is the only link to understanding for the public at large. This is frustrating. I would prefer not having to use the term at all.

And Michael:

If people come up to me and ask why I have all these lumps and bumps, I say, "Oh, this is called neurofibromatosis." Then I say, "Did you ever see 'The Elephant Man'?" If they say they did, then I tell them that I have what he had only he had a very extreme case and I only have little lumps and bumps and that there is a skin one and a bone one and I have the skin one and it isn't contagious. They can't catch it by sitting next to me or by drinking out of the same cup, and that one can only be born with it.

STIGMA

Affected persons and their families reported various kinds of fallout from the stigma connected with the condition. For family members this constituted "courtesy stigma," briefly mentioned by Goffman as the stigma that family and close associates of stigmatized persons may experience (Goffman 1963:30). For example, one subject reported that she went to her public library to find out what she could about NF1. As she tried to determine how to spell the word a librarian came over and asked if he could help her. She told him, "I think my child may have The Elephant Man's Disease. Could you help me find something on this?" He did find something she could read. She noticed that when she left the library all of the librarians were standing at the desk and staring at her. She decided then that she had better not say anything to anyone else about it.

Although the rediagnosis was made in 1986 (Tibbles and Cohen 1986), and since popularized (Newsweek 1988), NF1 is still at times associated with The Elephant Man in the media. When the discovery of the gene for NF1 occurred in 1990, television accounts and newspapers across the country labeled NF1 as "The Elephant Man's Disease."

The rediagnosis necessitated NF1's separation from the condition of The Elephant Man. However, because of the courage and dignity displayed by Joseph Merrick, it was difficult to simply walk away from that haunting image. For many, the memory of his dignity and character is as persistent as that of his shocking physical appearance. This consideration is expressed in the formal rediagnosis statement by Dr. John C. Carey in the National Neurofibromatosis Foundation newsletter, which reflected the significant humanistic issues involved in the rediagnosis:

None of this [necessity of making correct diagnosis] is meant to take anything away from the lessons that Mr. Merrick taught us. He is truly a study in human dignity and a prototype of an individual who can help us understand how people deal with uncertainty and disability. I hope that his diagnosis will continue to help honor his memory. I would certainly like to emphasize that the Foundation is not separating itself at all from the memory of this beautiful man, but only making sure that people with NF and people who are interested in his history know the correct medical diagnosis. (Carey 1988)

Within a context of unpredictability the specter of The Elephant Man as role model has served as a source of severe anxiety and depression for many subjects. Yet The Elephant Man also brought to the scientific quest many benefits often unknown to affected persons. The phenomenon of The Elephant Man may be seen as a bright meteor that flashed across the Western sky, attracting great public attention, rarely encountered congressional interest, and the blessings of funding, but leaving in its wake a conflictful two-fold legacy. While contributing significantly to scientific advances hailed as among the most dramatic and rapid known to modern science, the vivid image of that unfortunate man also precipitated fantasies evoking dread and horror for many affected persons and their families.

12

---

*Stigma**

The foregoing chapters reflect the pervasive force of stigma, society's obvious and expressed negative evaluation of their physical appearance or behavior, in essentially every area of many subjects' lives. Stigma is a daily companion for a great many persons whose NF1 is recognizable to the world. This chapter will report on the creation of stigma, its manifestations in the staring and comments of the general public, and how subjects thought about and dealt with these societal responses.

Isabelle, a sensitive and articulate older subject, now a quadriplegic as a result of spinal tumors and subsequent surgeries, described this irony of her life:

When I was in school I was really a good writer. I had an imagination, wrote stories about circus freaks, being in a freak show, in a circus, what that life was like even though I had never met a circus freak. The stories were so real that people thought I had actually talked to one or known one. It is funny; I look back at those stories and didn't know then at all about neurofibroma. I had no idea about The Elephant Man, but one story I wrote was about a woman who was horribly disfigured and was a circus freak. Her face was all swollen and cockeyed, her nose and her eyes were all to one side and her mouth was crooked. People would pay to come see her and see what her life was like, what she was like inside. That's the story I wrote and I was only fifteen years old. And when I read the story out loud everybody in the class cried, and they said they had never heard anything so sad in their life. And my teacher was totally blown away. I can remember the conversation because it stuck with me. He said, "Well, do you know someone like this?" I said, "No, I had never known anybody in my life like that, but I just thought about what it would be like to be so horribly ugly that people would pay to come see you and how awful that would be."

---

*Portions of this chapter are reprinted from Joan Ablon, Coping with Visible and Invisible Stigma: Neurofibromatosis 1, *In* Accessing the Issues: Current Research in Disability Studies, Elaine Makas, Beth Haller, and Tanis Doe, eds., pp. 45–49. Lewiston, ME: Society for Disability Studies and the Edmund S. Muskie Institute of Public Affairs, 1998. Reprinted with permission.

It is very pathetic, I guess, that that would happen to me. But I must have known somewhere that people would be staring at me someday. And when the doctor told me about The Elephant Man and the neurofibroma I flashed back to my story. I thought, "Oh, that's the story I wrote; it's going to be me; I'm going to be in the circus." That's the first thing I thought—"I'm going to be in the circus." I told Dr. Simmons that because he asked me, "What are you thinking about now that I have told you this. What are you thinking?" I said, "I'm going to be in the circus and people will pay to come look at me." And he said no one had ever given him an answer like that. But that's what I thought, that I could make a living by joining a circus, by being a geek.

The heterogeneity of presentation of NF1 creates a wide variety of possible symptoms ranging from visible stigmata of tumors on the skin, skeletal abnormalities, and optic gliomas, to the invisible ones of learning disabilities and the inability to reproduce without the possibility of passing on the condition to one's children. While most persons who have skin tumors experience them chiefly, and sometimes only, on the torso on areas that can be hidden by street dress, older persons and women past the age of childbearing often have them on the face, neck, and hands. Because scolioses and pseudoarthroses develop in early childhood, these can be visible from early ages on. The braces that children with these problems must often wear are also visible at times. Optic gliomas likewise develop early and their effects may be very visible from childhood on. While these objective physical symptoms of NF1 may be clearly apparent, the subjective experiencing of these and the social problems that may attend them vary. Learning disabilities tend to be manifest throughout the school and employment career and their consequences may likewise be variable. Feelings of stigma relating to the challenges of childbirth and/or the choice not to have children are even more difficult to gauge.

Clearly a great many persons with NF1 live with stigma as a daily companion. Twenty-nine, or more than one-half of the adult subjects brought up issues and problems in their lives that clearly fall under the rubric of stigma. While many of these persons would be classified within the more extreme categories of visibility and sometimes severity, almost equal numbers would fall into categories of mildly and moderately visible.

My drawing out and analyzing individuals' feelings of censorship by society and their remembrances of painful social interactions based on this censorship emphasize to me how the experiences of NF1 are always situated within the context of other issues of childhood and adulthood and also within specific personalities. While this fact makes it difficult or sometimes even impossible to compare the specific and ultimate meanings of stigma in differing cases, a general similarity in feelings of vulnerability and frustration is apparent.

THE CREATION OF STIGMA

Accounts of early stigmatization reflect that stigma is created and perpetuated through a number of social sources: most commonly by taunts of other children in school and the neighborhood, by the family, by doctors and medical personnel, and through the larger contexts of public opinion and values, media representations, and impersonal social interactions.

School was the primary childhood context for the development and maintenance of stigma. Academic and social challenges of school were often daunting, and as children, subjects frequently felt they were both academic and social failures in the eyes of their teachers and fellow schoolmates. Many of their accounts were presented in Chapter 5.

Family as Generators of Stigma

In five cases the behavior of parents or other family members instilled in the subjects as children the fact they had a "terrible" and "shameful" condition. Subjects report that the families in these instances were all "dysfunctional" or "unhappy," and the presence of a genetically affected child became the lightning rod for problems and abuse of various kinds. The affected children grew up in cocoons of shame and misery, which are reflected in their unhappiness and emotional problems as adults. Terry spoke bitterly of the creation of the stigma around her condition by parents who never put a name to it, telling her that something bad was very wrong with her, but that she should not complain about her symptoms:

I was a scared spirit. That's a spirit that is very, very afraid, because I was born flawed and I was reminded of it everyday of my life. Never told about my disease but always told in other ways that I was flawed. And there was always something wrong with me, and I think my disease just complicated it. I think it might have happened anyway, but I think my disease made a major contribution and complication.

Sarah talked about her early physical abuse in her family and her role as the scapegoat for family problems. These exacerbated visible symptoms of NF1 and resulted in a cycle of abuse that now, even in her thirties, she cannot leave behind.

When I was growing up I'd be called "ugly," by the kids. They would say I was a freak. I would go home and cry and my family would tell me that there was nothing wrong with me, to just ignore it. But I was also physically abused there. Me and my parents would argue and they were getting divorced and I became the responsible party in my eyes. So I would go back to school and it would be the same old cycle, on and on.

One husband of a very visibly affected woman told me that her family's behavior to the present day reflects their shame at her condition. "They still don't want her around. When she went to visit them in Fresno they took her to a restaurant nine miles out of town, and not for the food, either."

Medical Personnel as Generators of Stigma

At least a dozen visibly affected adults spoke of behaviors of doctors and other medical personnel that they found stigmatizing. Not only did these behaviors reflect that medical personnel thought negatively of their condition but they also bore a message that the person affected with NF1 should be ashamed of it. Said Harry:

I don't like using the word, but I've been a "genetic freak" for a long time to doctors. That's the way I feel about it. I don't like the word "genetic" and I don't like the word "freak," but that's what you feel like after a while. You walk into a hospital, and they'll come charging at you. Then after they see how hard my case is they don't want anything to do with me. I think from the time I was six years old all the way through, I was more or less an exhibit for every doctor who wanted something to look at. I was a freak show, I guess. I'm that term, that's about it. I was a genetic wonder, a genetic oddity.

Maureen recounted an episode that had happened to her at a large regional hospital:

I was with my husband, and we went to have some blood drawn, and the lab technician said, "Oooo, are you contagious or what do you have?" My heart dropped. Because here I am, you know, thinking, "Oh life's cool; life's easy; let's go get the blood drawn and we'll go have lunch." So the next time that I had to go and get blood drawn, after one time and something like this has happened, when you have to go again you think, "I don't want to do this. Somebody might say that again." Now I can understand that people are ignorant, but for somebody in the health profession?

Norita bitterly described an episode that happened in a Central American country when she was applying for her U.S. citizenship papers:

They picked out the doctor you have to go to. I went to the doctor and he asked me to undress and he weighed me and everything. Then he said, "What's this that you have?" I said, "Neurofibromatosis." He asked if I went to swimming pools and to the beach and I told him I did, and I asked him why he asked. He said, "Aren't you ashamed?" I said, "Excuse me?" I had gone to swimming pools and I had gone to the beach. It didn't bother me. Well, okay, it *did* bother me when people stared. But I went anyhow. But after this it was worse. He started really putting me down. He said I should be ashamed. I said, "But this is not contagious. It's genetic."

AMERICAN COSMETIC VALUES AND MEDIA REPRESENTATIONS

Many persons brought up the import of the mass media in influencing, shaping, and clearly demonstrating strict and far-reaching American cosmetic values. Women tended to be more bitter in their comments than men. Said Annie:

I can be very self-conscious of my skin condition to the point where I think, I wouldn't sit here in my bathing suit. On TV and in commercials, you see all these bathing beauties, where you have the picture perfect skin, you know, the 36-24-36 figure. So that when you'll see these commercials for acne, you think, "So here you are with somebody that's so upset because they have a pimple on their face, and I have this all over me." Society puts a label on you that if you don't have a clear complexion, there is something wrong with you.

The impact of "The Elephant Man" was discussed in Chapter 11. Mention of The Elephant Man, believed for some eighty years to have had NF1, was frequently made throughout the interviews. Most persons felt that the association with The Elephant Man has contributed to the stigma around NF1. My conversations with subjects about the stigma surrounding The Elephant Man precipitated a number of vehement statements from them about the stigma around physical difference and disability. Said Harry's girlfriend:

Harry called me and said, "Come over, there's a movie I want you to see." We sat on the bed watching "The Elephant Man" on TV. I cried. I said, "No man should be treated like that," and I cried and cried. Harry said, "That's what I'm considered, a freak." I said, "You're no freak, you're a man."

Harry: Society doesn't tolerate physical difference. I do know that right now we're in a transition where the disabled are going back in the closet.

What do you think is causing that?

Society. If anybody like Joseph Merrick lived today, he'd have the same problem. Anybody with deformities will not be able to exist in society. The sixties and the early seventies were the decades of changes. That's when things were a hell of a lot better than we have them now. I think the attitude now is like we're back in the fifties again. I don't think different looking people in the world will ever be accepted out in public. I don't think that time will come. I think severe deformities, severe disabilities will always be hidden in the closet away from the public. Even though you can have all the intelligence in the world, you can be a genius, but if you're deformed, if you're in a wheelchair, or have a disability, you'll be hidden. There will never come a time when The Elephant Man will ever be accepted in society. It won't happen in 2,000 years. Never.

And Isabelle:

I think what the movie "The Elephant Man" wanted to do it didn't do at all. I think it's ridiculous. What it's supposed to do is make people feel compassionate and good toward people that have these grotesque things and are different than they are. But it only works while they are in the movie. I watched other people, and they would get tears in their eyes and they'd say, "Oh, I feel so sorry for him, and why do they treat him like that?" But those very people, when they left the theater, if they had to run into somebody that looked like that, they would run away in terror or turn their faces. Only while they're in the movie do they think differently. Like Jerry's kids, once a year he parades all those little pathetic kids out in their wheelchairs and people feel sorry for them and they write out checks and they send the money, and they say, "Oh, when I see a person in a wheelchair, I'm going to be nicer," but they're not. It doesn't do any good; it doesn't change people's attitudes. People are never going to change. When I go out in my wheelchair, people just wish I wasn't around. Horace insists on taking me to nice restaurants, real nice restaurants where everybody's all dressed up and everything's real fancy, and I come rolling in in my wheelchair and people don't like it.

Why do you think that?

I can tell. And I'm not being paranoid, and I'm not being unfair. People feel uncomfortable around somebody in a wheelchair. Especially since I have to be fed. I can't feed myself. I do look nice when I go out. Horace fixes my hair beautifully. He puts on my make-up and I wear beautiful clothes that I had before I got sick, and we go into this real nice restaurant. So you see a woman all dressed up and then I have to be fed. And it just makes people uncomfortable.

But I'm a hypocrite in a lot of ways because I'm the same way myself. There's certain people I see in wheelchairs that make me uncomfortable. People that I don't want to be around. So I think that I'm not any different than the people I condemn.

And Nathan:

A lot of times I would talk with my cancer support group about NF. A lot of them have been through it, because cancer and NF are very similar in a lot of ways. Cancer is a little far along. A lot of people now don't believe you can catch cancer, whereas they used to. They would think you can just catch NF like the flu or something. But it's a lot of the similar problems of dealing with disfigurement and people's stereotypes of how you should or shouldn't be.

And Sarah:

It depends on *how* we are different as to whether we are acceptable to society or not. For example, look at dwarfs. They are only short. As long as they are cute dwarfs then people can look very charitable by treating people who are different looking as equals. Very often they are almost looked at as children. "They're precious; they're cute." However, this attitude could almost be as debilitating, in a way, because they are not treated as adults.

If people see someone in a wheelchair they tend to treat that person with some sort of compassion because their difference is visual. It can be seen and it can be seen that something happened to that person. Whereas a person who is disfigured in some manner but isn't in a wheelchair or in some other way indicates that he or she has been in an accident, and that there are no heroics involved, then I think that the public attitude becomes quite different.

Many subjects noted that the only person or few persons they had ever seen with NF1 were very visibly affected persons on television. Such persons, no doubt, were typically chosen for talk shows because of their dramatic appearance. While engaging the interest of the general public, such representation ordinarily frightens affected persons who do not know the limits to which their own condition might progress. For example, Randy stated that the sudden and dramatic appearance of tumors on the face and hands of a doctor on the television program "L.A. Law" was the basis for his fear of tumors rapidly growing on his face in middle age.

EXPERIENCING AND COPING WITH STIGMA IN EVERYDAY LIFE

Each person works out his or her own modes of coping or struggling with stigma. Many persons talked about their problems in accepting the way they look, or in accepting the shame caused by the negative responses of others.

The following two statements describe differing responses to basically similar problems of two very different women—Harriet, a middle-aged, white grandmother who lives in the suburbs, and Carrie, an African American of early middle age and also a grandmother, from the inner city of a metropolitan area. Both of these women were the second generation of NF1-affected women in their families. Said Harriet:

I mean, how often can you say that you feel bad because of the way you look and that you are not able to accept it? I feel real angry at myself for not accepting myself when there are things that other people have that are worse than what I have. I can see; I can function; I can work. But this society is based on how we look. I mean everything is. Not what we are, but how we look.

I would think that I am able to bury it pretty well and sometimes, even when I'm looking in the mirror, I can bury it enough to think, "Well, you know, I'm not unattractive." I tell myself that so that I don't, for one thing, feel sorry for myself and think how ugly I am and repulsive. And there's times I look in the mirror and put on my make-up but not see myself. I'm not seeing anybody else; I've not seen a perfect image; I'm not saying that. I'm just saying that I'm looking in the mirror and not looking. I think it's hard for most people to be able to perceive themselves, because you may have whatever image you have, it may not have to do with what you're seeing. I sort of have a hard time with my sister in this way. She has a lot of self-confidence and she's more outgoing. I would say that I'm real introverted. I'm drawing more and more into a shell. Sometimes it's very hard for me to go out at all.

Harriet turned her concerns about her appearance inward, with her depression causing considerable unhappiness and inability to take advantage of possible sources of pleasure in life. Carrie, on the other hand, rebelled against the negative responses to her appearance. Said Carrie:

Like, it bothers me not being able to wear short sleeves because it looks very bad. I was like real self-conscious about it. So, I started getting all the surgeries done. And the more I got done, the less I started feeling self-conscious about it because that was a big thing for years.

Being self-conscious?

Yes, because in New York you look like a junkie with bandages and shit. And I was like covering up with band aids. It was, "You donated blood?" "Yeah," because it was an easy thing to say. When I was out in the street I kept it covered and didn't roll up my sleeves past the bandage and that went on for a long time. I went through thousands of band aids doing that because I just did not want anybody to see it. It really looked gross. And if it looked gross to me, it had to look gross to somebody else. I couldn't deal with it at all. I just could not go out looking like that. So, before I came out here I started getting everything done, to where it doesn't look so bad anymore. Also I started thinking, "To hell with it, if I want to wear short sleeves or go out like I am, I will."

Did you ever say anything in New York, I mean in the subway or elsewhere if anybody stared?

Basically, I said, "What the hell you looking at? What's your problem?"

And would they say anything?

Nothing. "Nothing wrong."

Staring: "What the Hell Are You Looking At?"

Most persons in discussing reactions of the public distinguished between the behavior and comments of children as opposed to those of adults. They acknowledge that children's questions and actions are more natural and understandable. Once a child is old enough to know better, then staring and rude questions are not appropriate behaviors. The following are a selection from a large array of examples given by subjects.

Said Marilee:

I would be at points too where I would forget what condition that I have. It'll be sometimes a small child that will bring it up. The last time I went to see a movie, I went to stand in line and a little kid freaked out and he said, "Mommy, mommy, chicken pox." That's a downer too. But you could understand a child, because children are very honest. But it's true, I could have a lot of anger or resentments that, "No, I'm not normal," and I could forget that I have this disfigurement, but yet a small child will bring me back to reality, that, "Yes, you do."

And Lou, a woman with a significant scoliosis:

I try to get clothes to maybe not show my back and how I walk, but sometimes I don't realize how I walk. Some people used to make fun of me. Adults are the worst. Sometimes it really does bother me and it makes me upset and other times I don't pay any attention.

A middle-aged affected woman recounted this story at an NF support group meeting to an outraged audience and later to me again in her home:

I had won a subscription to a health club, and I went to the club and they showed me all around. I was to come back the next day to sign the contract. The next morning before I left, I got a phone call from the health club saying that they would prefer that I not come back. Whatever I had was unsightly and would frighten other people away, and not to come back till I was cured. That was really the worst thing that had ever happened to me.

Private Issues Made Public

Several persons gave accounts of being rudely accosted by strangers who were curious about their condition, or who wished to comment on their symptoms. Said Rachel:

Several years ago before I had the tumors around my hips removed I was just in constant, constant pain. I had the flaps and the folds. And they were all around my hips. And people would think I was pregnant. Strangers would come up to me on the street. And they would ask me when the baby was due. And if you desperately want to have children as much as I do, and you desperately know that you can't have them, I find those questions very, very hard.

I used to feel invaded as a child. When I used to walk around with a body brace, or a body cast, people would stop me on the street and ask me what was wrong. And, I felt invaded. I felt like I was being raped. Strangers! Strangers would ask me. So, I would make up stories. I would tell people I fell off a skateboard going down Lombard Street. I mean, it was none of their business. And no one, no one has the right to do that to a child. I don't care what good intentions the world has. No one has a right, a stranger especially, to ask a child anything.

Explaining Their Condition

The great majority of subjects reported that if asked they explained NF1 by referring to "The Elephant Man's Disease" since this is a publicly known condition but "neurofibromatosis" is a long, unpronounceable, and obscure term. Most stated they would make it clear that while The Elephant Man had a very serious and dramatic case of NF1, their case was mild. About half stated they amended their explanation to say the condition was no longer related to The Elephant Man. A variety of other explanations of NF1 were also reported. Said Rudy:

When people do ask, what do you tell them?

It depends. If it's an adult and they're curious and concerned, no problem. I'll spend as much time as need be. If they're really abrasive about it, I'll cut them off. It's on a case-by-case basis. As for kids, a lot of times it's normally about my eye. "Is there any eye in there?" and I'll say, "No." And they'll swallow it. For the real little ones, I bend on down and take off the glasses and I say, "You know, there's no eye in there," and I'll lean closer to them so they can see, and a lot of times, right there they won't ask questions. But if they do, they say, "Why did you take it out?" and I'll explain, "Well, see one of these, see these bumps here, there was one on the eye, and it was no good."

And Robbie:

It gets very tiring having to explain over and over and over and over again, particularly that the only way I can give it to someone is if I'm their father, and do it genetically. You can't catch blue eyes from someone. Or another thing people always are saying is they know how to cure it. "Oh, take this vitamin; eat this way; stop eating that." And then having to bite your tongue and tell them, "You can't cure blue eyes." They think it's something they can easily cure with vitamins. I try to explain that all that has been tried for a few hundred years. It's genetic. You can't change chromosomes at this point.

One very visibly affected woman at an NF support group meeting stated:

Oh! I don't have any problems with children. I just tell all of the kids that God loves me so much, that he loves me with every one of these tumors. Every tumor that I have tells me that He loves me more. The kids would say, "Oh, how can I get those tumors? I want tumors."

Rachel talked about the pervading affects of comments and stares on her consciousness:

How this sense of stigma is played out in my life is my commitment to left-wing politics. If anyone would ask me what are the positive aspects of having NF, I would say that they are two-fold. One is, I know what it is like to be a "nigger" in society. I know what it's like to be the leper. I know what it is to be judged for your appearance and not your ability. And, because of that, I really am committed to building a society where these issues aren't going to be thrown in people's faces. I think because I grew up genetically challenged and disabled that my commitment is stronger.

I know what it is to see prejudice. I experience people judging me because of the way I look. And that angers me. And so, if there is any aspect of NF that was positive, it is this. I mean, it's a hell of a way to be politically conscious!

13

NF Support Groups

Two major foundations exist to promote and fund scientifically reviewed research, to provide information and support for individuals and families affected by both NF1 and NF2, and to educate professionals and the general public. The National Neurofibromatosis Foundation, Inc. (NNFF) has thirty-two chapters over the country. The NNFF has promoted and funded most of the research that led to the localization and subsequent isolation of the NF1 gene, and has also funded at least one major meeting annually where scientists and clinicians working on NF1 gene research can exchange findings. This foundation also sponsors local support groups, medical conferences, and a very successful summer camp for affected teenagers.

Neurofibromatosis, Inc. (NF, Inc.), has nine chapters, chiefly on the east coast, in the midwest, Arizona, and Mississippi. NF, Inc. also promotes and funds research, and sponsors national and local conferences and educational forums. Like the NNFF, NF, Inc. prints and distributes educational materials for affected persons and professionals. NF, Inc. has been particularly concerned with patient support activities and sponsors many support groups and short-term therapy groups led by genetic counselors and social workers. A number of independent local support groups also exist in Texas, Florida, Michigan, Oklahoma, and California. See Appendix IV for addresses of the foregoing resources.

NF support group meetings sponsored by the NNFF and the California Neurofibromatosis Network, which was in existence in the late 1980s, were held in three geographic areas of northern California during the research period. The occurrence of meetings varied between areas with meetings held typically two or three times a year. The volunteer coordinators made arrangements for meetings and carried out other NF-related activities, fitting these into their own busy and hectic work and family schedules. Coordinators also recruited members to participate in the Human Race, an annual fundraising activity, as well as other fundraising events.

The NNFF and the California Neurofibromatosis Network both sponsored a number of full-day medical conferences in the Los Angeles and San Francisco Bay areas during the research period. These informational events targeted both health professionals and laypersons and featured talks by medical specialists, panel discussions, and workshops on diverse issues. The audiences for these conferences typically numbered from 100 to 200 hundred persons.

The regional coordinators receive many telephone calls from parents of newly diagnosed children, from adults who also may be newly diagnosed, and from health care professionals such as genetic counselors who wish to refer clients. Lay callers are often referred by agencies such as the Easter Seal Society and by doctors or genetic counselors. One coordinator reported that the calls often come in unevenly, but receiving three to four calls a week would not be unusual. Coordinators report that few of the lay people who call for information actually come to support group meetings or medical conferences. Anxiety caused by fear of meeting others with the condition and denial appear to be important factors in inhibiting the actual attendance of those who call for information about meetings.

FIRST ENCOUNTERS

Approximately two-thirds of the subjects had attended at least one NF support group meeting or educational conference, and one-third of these attended meetings with some regularity. Subjects reported a broad range of avenues that first led them to the NNFF and the California Neurofibromatosis Network and then on to attendance at support groups meetings and medical conferences. In fact, subjects learned about the organizations and group meetings through twenty-two differing modes, the chief ones being: talk shows or informational spot announcements on television (often in conjunction with a showing of "The Elephant Man") which they, their relatives, or friends saw; magazine articles; information from others with NF1 who approached them and told them about local meetings of the organizations; or referral by doctors or personnel at genetics programs. The statements below reflect the diversity of these often circuitous modes of learning about the organizations:

My wife heard about it. Linda's [the coordinator's] neighbor was xeroxing some NF materials for her at the bank where my wife Amy works and Amy saw them and she said to me when she came home, "Hey, there's this foundation for NF and they have a meeting at the hospital next Sunday. Do you want to go?"

One of the ladies at one of the jobsites where I worked has NF. She noticed my bumps. "Do you have neurofibromatosis?" she said to me one day. I told her I did. "Do you know there's this group where you can get information?" I said, "No." She told me that the next time she came in she would bring me information and she did.

My doctor asked me had I ever done any research into NF. I said, "No." I'd never even thought about researching NF. "Well, you're a researcher. You're an academic. Get on with it! You can find out answers to your questions just as well as I can." And it was a real good response, because it made me take responsibility. There is something called the *Directory of Organizations*. And I looked up NF and there it was. I'd never even heard about this organization before. They were in New York and I wrote them.

Less than ten persons heard about the NNFF or the California Neurofibromatosis Network and their activities from their doctors or from the genetics department of a hospital they had consulted. Fortunately this situation is improving. A major effort of the NNFF has been professional education of doctors nationally through the distribution of informational packets and medical conferences carrying continuing education credits. The Foundation also staffs booths at medical specialty conventions.

First Reactions

Subjects recounted numerous reactions to their first support group meeting. The most common reaction was a feeling of relief at meeting others who shared their condition. For example:

When you feel that you are very different, and you look very different, and you think you're about the only person out there with it, it is a comfort to know that you are not by yourself, that there are other people out there that you can share with, or that they can share with you.

Some said that the fear of seeing severely affected persons was their first reaction:

I was very frightened to go in because I didn't know what I'd see or what degree of handicap I'd see. Outwardly, you don't know I have it. So, I was kind of curious to see how other people with NF looked. It wasn't so bad. I mean, I don't have it that bad and I couldn't imagine what someone who had it bad would look like. I was thinking that someone would look like The Elephant Man. It's a little frightening to see. But you couldn't tell people had it, either. I think I was afraid to see someone that might have had it worse than me and think, "My God, there but by the grace of God go I."

Several persons stated that seeing others worse off than themselves had, in fact, made them feel better about their own condition. Said Theresa:

You feel strange and you don't know what you're going to experience when you get there. But you feel better about yourself, I think, because, especially at the university, people come from all over. You might think that we're bad off, and then you see other people, someone worse than us, and someone's worse than them; there's always someone worse off. You count your blessings when you go there.

We were not aware really about how serious it can be until we started going to these meetings at Crawford and then I was appalled. We've been very fortunate that we haven't experienced the things that some of the people we've met there have experienced. I think if I was from this generation and if I knew then what I've learned now, I really would have been very hesitant about having a family. God, if you knew you were going to bring a child into the world that might suffer some of the things that some of these people that we've met there have suffered, it would be taking a real responsibility. But I guess, ignorance is bliss, because I didn't know.

Others described a variety of reactions evoked by comparing the conditions and life situations of those whom they saw there to their own. Said Rachel:

I remember going to my first meeting and coming home and just crying. There were three women there with NF besides myself. Of the four of us, three were unmarried and didn't seem to have any special person in their life. One woman had the most amazing man with her. This man loved her. This man knew about the NF and he didn't care. And he was up front. He said, "I love this woman and this is her issue and I'm here because her issue is my issue." And I was so impressed because he loved her. He was there for her. And I was so incredibly envious of her.

I came home and cried because they were my sisters and my brothers and I had been denied access to them all my life. I cried for that little baby whose parents seemed to be just awash with fear. And they didn't know quite how to put everything together. And, I cried because I have NF and I hate it. I wish I could change it. I wish I had a wonderful life. I wish I did not have a genetic disease. And I cried for the babies I'll never have. I really found it very stressful. Cathartic and stressful.

SUBJECTS' EVALUATION OF MEETINGS

Meetings were essentially of two formats, informational/speaker meetings and sharing/discussions. Speaker meetings featured a professional with clinical or educational expertise who spoke and answered questions. Speakers were most commonly geneticists but might be dermatologists, genetic counselors, other clinical specialists who see children, or specialists on learning disorders or speech problems, which a great many children with NF1 manifest. Following the speaker, a discussion or sharing of experiences over coffee and refreshments takes place. Sharing/discussion meetings were those in which members talked about their own experiences and problems in more detail and how they dealt with these, again typically over refreshments.

The attitudes of affected adults about meetings and their assessments of their utility varied as widely as their symptoms and other characteristics, yet were not correlated with these. Neither severity nor visibility predicted the opinions about the usefulness or the value of the meetings. Gender appeared to be somewhat predictive, with five men stating they would not attend support groups at all. However, other men did attend meetings and found the meetings useful. Speaker meetings were almost universally well accepted and considered to be valuable because most persons came to meetings for information. However, opinions varied widely about the utility of discussion groups, with men and women equally positive and negative about them.

The same split in opinions was present in the global evaluations of meetings. For instance, this positive evaluation from a woman:

The most important thing for me was understanding some of the things that had happened in my life, like my early development. I was thrilled when I heard of things I had gone through that were typical for people who had NF. That was nice. I was no longer a freak because those things had happened. I could close that chapter in my life.

In contrast this opinion from a man:

Did you find out anything from the talks or meetings?

Yeah, give me a shot and get it over with. Be completely cured, that would be fine. I might go down and do that. But I'm essentially not interested. What good would it do? What would it change? The next morning everything would still be the same. I still wouldn't be able to reach up to the second shelf.

Most local speaker and discussion meeting focused on problems of children. Nonaffected parents of affected children were more in evidence at meetings than were adults with NF. Many of the adults who had attended meeting commented to me that they felt they would have benefited more from groups that focused chiefly on concerns of adults. Also some persons stated that they found the discussions about children's problems depressing because these brought back memories of their own childhood problems. Said Rhoda, reflecting on her dismal school history, "Basically, we want our own thing. We've already gone through those things once. I don't need to relive it."

MEMBERS WHO DO NOT ATTEND MEETINGS

Many persons, and proportionately more male subjects, belong to the NNFF and receive their newsletters and other materials but do not wish to go to support group meetings because they do not feel they need "support" (see Chapter 9). Several persons stated that they do not go to meetings because they are too fearful of seeing others worse than themselves with a condition that they might one day share. For example, said Terry:

I wouldn't even have talked with anyone else with NF up until a couple of months ago. I couldn't go to the groups. I knew the groups were happening but I couldn't go. I couldn't be around somebody who might be worse than I am; couldn't look at somebody who I might be like one day. I couldn't do it. And I don't know if I can now. I think I need to start talking to people on some level about it, because if I don't, I know for me it will never get resolved and it will never get healed and I'll keep being angry.

The logistics of attending meetings that often were geographically distant were discouraging to some. Three persons stated they did not drive or had physical problems that made a one-hour drive to a meeting impossible. Others stated they could not spare the time from busy work schedules and family responsibilities to attend a meeting that might require, including transportation, a four- or five-hour time commitment.

The variety of experiences with and attitudes toward NF meetings reported by subjects was in keeping with the variety of presentations of NF1 and the life experiences of subjects themselves. What is clear however, is the overriding value of having available major foundations which support education and research. I was struck by the lack of knowledge of the persons I interviewed who were not associated with nor on the mailing lists of the foundations. Consequently, they had no way of learning about recent developments around their condition. For example, most of these persons had no knowledge of the rediagnosis of The Elephant Man's Disease even five years or longer after the fact. While the diversity of NF1 as it is experienced challenges a common generic support group goal of building "we-ness," that is, a sense of community, the foundations serve affected individuals in numerous and diverse manners even though the ultimate goal of these organizations, that of finding a cure, may take a number of years more to achieve.

14

Medical Experiences

Elise observed during one of our many hours of discussing medical care:

Doctors tell people terrible things because they lack information and also lack compassion. Medicine is not a compassionate profession. There are certain areas that they don't see as life threatening or as a big problem for them. But they are not the ones who have to live with it.

Thirty-three affected adults commented on the quality of their medical care (exclusive of psychotherapy) as they related their medical histories. Of six who were also parents of affected children, four tended to be more focused on their children's care than their own. Because of the numerous specialists that many affected children see in addition to their pediatrician or internist, parents' worries and time expenditures around their children's care were highlighted rather than their own NF1-related and general health concerns.

The largest number of affected adults, eighteen, described their health care as a mixture of good and bad experiences. Eight others said that their care was mostly good or excellent. Three persons of these eight commented on the need to be aggressive or ever-vigilant to receive good care. Three persons stated their care was all good, and four stated their medical experiences were essentially all negative. Many subjects were currently seeing helpful and sensitive doctors and contrasted their current positive experiences to very negative ones in their past that they would likely never forget. In most cases evaluations were based not on poor clinical care, but on doctors' dramatic statements or behavior that subjects considered rude, insensitive, or unnecessarily frightening.

Many subjects bear the brunt of having to juggle seeing many different doctors—internists, dermatologists, neurologists, ophthalmologists, or orthopedists.

Subjects reported their experiences with numerous health care systems that they had to negotiate, often with considerable difficulty. One-half of the affected adults belong to a large health maintenance organization (HMO) identified herein as Harper Hospital. Most had chosen Harper because it was the least expensive option, particularly if they had children. Patients often had little choice of the doctors they saw at Harper. Typically, they waited for long periods to be seen by a doctor and often instead saw nurse practitioners. About one-half felt satisfied or noncommittal about their services at Harper Hospital. The rest often angrily told tales of being treated cursorily or even with poor clinical care.

Other health insurance included other HMOs, Blue Cross, programs for armed service veterans and their dependents, other private programs, and Medicare or Medi-Cal if persons were receiving disability, unemployment benefits, or were sixty-five and over. Under a number of these programs the choices of doctors often were very circumscribed, and even if subjects heard of more appropriate doctors they could not seek out their services. Lou, who had a severe scoliosis, had been operated on numerous times by the same master orthopedic surgeon and treated by a sympathetic internist from her childhood years. She was informed that because of a change in medical policy, her treatment by these doctors would not be covered henceforth by her health insurance because they did not practice in the county in which she lived. With difficulty she continued to see them and pay for her visits out of a very marginal budget.

Persons with NF1, as with other genetic conditions, ordinarily had to rely on group policies to cover their health needs because their NF1 would be categorized as a "preexisting condition" and hence not coverable under an individual policy. Several stayed in poor paying or highly unsatisfying jobs because they were afraid of leaving their health insurance programs. An example is Jim, who spoke with me in detail about his financial problems as a low-paid security guard with minimal health benefits. Many of his experiences mirror the dilemmas of other subjects:

The last time I went to the doctor was four years ago. He gave me $100 worth of medicine and I couldn't afford the medicine. My plan doesn't pay for medicines. I went to the druggist and I told him what I needed and asked how much it cost before he prepared it. He said, "$125." That was for two little bottles of medicine. I didn't get it. I had a choice between this one and Harper, and Harper doesn't have a dental plan and I have bad teeth. I needed to have dental coverage and Harper doesn't offer it.

THE GOOD DOCTORS

While medical competency was important to all subjects, female subjects who described their satisfaction with their doctors also tended to emphasize that their doctors cared about them as individuals, were thoughtful of them, and sensitive to their concerns. Theresa recounted:

As far as doctors are concerned, I've had the same doctor all these years. I haven't had any bad experiences with doctors, because Dr. White is very compassionate and a very nice man. I've just stuck with him all these years. I go to him because he gives the pap smears and the blood work and because I'm—how can I say it—I'm comfortable with him. I trust him and he's been very good to me, like, he's that kind of doctor.

Years ago I was at some bad point in our lives. It was just really a horrendous time and Dr. White would see me after office hours and he'd counsel me and it was like no charge or anything like that. Mostly what it was, I talked and cried a lot. And then he'd pose a question to me, "Well now, what do you think you should be doing about this, Theresa?" He's unique.

And Norita:

I didn't want a woman doctor. I used to think she will criticize, or maybe I would be jealous because of her smooth skin. But Dr. Apperson, I just happen to like her. I went with my guards up when I went to see her. I was ready to fight her. And then she's so sweet. I couldn't do anything. And I thought, "Well, if I don't like her, I don't have to see her again." But she was so sweet, so nice. I talked to her over the phone and then I went to see her. What it is with me, she has been so kind and so caring, it's like she knows me as a person and not just this number that comes in and goes out. She remembers what we talked about the time before and all that. And having what I have, I have been with a lot of doctors, and no one has done that. I adore her.

And Lou:

Dr. Rabin knows all my little things, and then with my back problem when he gives me a pap smear he screams for the nurse to bring in three pillows to put my back up so I don't hurt myself. And he says, "Get those pillows for her; she needs those pillows!" I just feel comfortable with him, so I just pay for it.

Sharon enthusiastically talked about her surgeon:

Dr. Jacobson was very responsive at the time of my surgery. My sisters and their husbands would come and we'd have this big conference because they wanted to ask all these questions. Once they were in his office, all five of us, and he said, "Is everybody here? Aren't there any more?" And they're all laughing. Every time he saw me in the hospital, as he left the room, he'd tweak my toe. When I left the hospital he hugged me. He didn't need to do that. He was always very nice and when any of my family called to ask questions he'd respond. He would call back immediately and spend a long time talking to them on the phone.

Male subjects tended to focus more on the functional aspects of their relationships with their doctors or on clinical competence. For example, said Ronald, "I think my care has been fine. But I don't know any better either. I have nothing to compare it to. I'm alive; I'm still getting around. I'm still able to drive, and function fairly well."

PATIENTS' COMPLAINTS

Involuntary Display

Many subjects bitterly commented that doctors treat them as curiosities. Some reported situations they regarded as voyeuristic. The most common complaint was that doctors who subjects had consulted brought in other doctors to look at their visible symptoms. Subjects agreed to this because they felt they had no other choice or because they were too shy to refuse. Recounted Theresa:

The doctor that delivered the baby, I still remember his name was Dr. Herald. He was just, how can I say it, very interested and very amazed and the day after I delivered the baby, he came in and he said to me, "You know, you have a very unusual condition here. And doctors can be doctors all their lives and they never see this condition that you have. Is it okay with you if I bring in a couple of doctors to see you?"

What do you do? You're a kid, you're twenty-one and you're gonna argue with this colonel or major? And I said, "Well, I guess it's okay." He left and came back with four other doctors and the hospital chaplain. I mean, I was like a specimen. And they were pointing to this one and then pointing to that one [tumors]. Just pointing at different things without any regard to how I might have felt, disrobed there, with people staring down at me. And they weren't very sensitive, you know, to maybe how I felt being discussed.

Victor angrily recalled this incident which reflects some of the specific issues around confidentiality that should be considered in a small community.

When I was eighteen, just out of school, I walked into an emergency ward with strep throat. Finally they said, "Hey, you have neurofibromas," and the doctor said a big long name and then he said, "Do you mind if I let people come in here and look at you?" I didn't even have a chance to say, "No," and he had people going in there and looking at me, including, mind you, the cleaning lady. I'm sitting there totally devastated. I couldn't handle it. One thing, it would be getting back to Sue, my wife. She was just my girlfriend, then. She knew I had it, but the cleaning lady was her aunt, who is very, I mean, she's Miss Prissy. There ain't no dust on her floor or nothing and here is someone who has been dating her niece, and mind you, he's got neurofibromas. She's thinking, "How am I going to break this to Sue?" Sue's aunt now knows everything about it. She knows it is inherited and that it is ugly and it can cause you to go blind.

The issue was they brought in Sue's relative, the cleaning lady. They had no business doing that. I didn't have the chance to say, "No." I was mad. My dad was in the waiting room and the doctor goes and tells my dad that I had a mental problem. "Your son's got a definite mental problem." He didn't tell him what he had done. Had he, my dad probably would have nailed him. Doctors need to be educated not to do that kind of thing. I didn't want everybody to know that I had it. Oh man, to this day if I go in there and that doctor is there, I don't want to mess with him. I don't know his name but I know him by sight and I've got him marked. I don't like people treating me like that, making me into a freak. Now I can talk about it, but I still don't want to be made into a spectacle: "Look at him!"

Yet, four other persons recounted that they had been displayed to other doctors but as adults that it had never bothered them. While in general women seemed to resent involuntary display more than men, one of these four was a woman. Reggie recalled:

I went before the tumor board at University Hospital. These doctors came from Switzerland, Spain, France, Europe, all over the place. They spoke very little English. Fine and dandy. It didn't bother me. When I was down there they also brought students around every day, eight to ten students a day to look at me. That didn't bother me because I figured, "Well, maybe one of these young people coming through will have the answers. So why not let them look? Why not let them poke? That's okay." Being on exhibition didn't bother me. I figured maybe this young doctor will have the answer some day.

Several persons expressed their ambivalence about not wanting to be stared at, while at the same time also knowing that medical practitioners must have the opportunity to learn about unusual health conditions. Sarah commented, "I know they have to be there to learn, and I am so glad they are there, but it is tough to be there with that. They draw lines on my face. They treat you like you are a specimen, talk about you like you are a hunk of meat."

Complaints and Concerns Ignored

As noted above, many subjects expressed their appreciation to doctors who took their condition and their concerns seriously. In contrast, others felt their symptoms and their fears and concerns about potentially serious problems related to their NF1 were ignored or trivialized. Said Julia, a woman who has numerous tumors on the face, neck, and hands:

It's like when someone comes in with a concern. For instance, let's say you've got these tumors on your face or something bothers you and you'd like to get it taken off. They won't take it off. They say, "Oh, that's not so bad." They are not the ones living with it. They tell you it's not serious. When a patient comes in and says something irritates them, the doctors should do something about it.

Many subjects report that doctors frequently refuse to remove external tumors unless they are large or become very uncomfortable even though the subjects find them unsightly or have other reasons why they want them removed. Doctors sometimes say at meetings that some tumors are highly vascular and might bleed a lot, or might grow back in a relatively short period of time. If doctors could clearly explain to patients their reasons for not wanting to remove certain tumors or carry out other procedures then patients could better understand the bases for doctors' decision-making and would be less likely to feel their wishes and concerns were ignored.

Negativity and Insensitive Statements

Many subjects complained about doctors' negativity and general insensitivity to them and their condition. Doctors made evident their negativity through general attitude, style of relating, and verbal messages. One of the most dramatic experiences was recalled bitterly by Rachel:

I have yet another medical horror story for the whole world to hear. That is, when I was fifteen my mother said, "You really do need a medical checkup. You're a young woman now and you need to see a teenage doctor." And she took me to an internist who was, as I'd call it, "a graduate of the Dachau School of Medicine!" He basically said, "You have NF. I think you should be sterilized because you shouldn't bring any more defective babies into the world." And at fifteen with my emerging sexuality, oh my, my! It was horrible. It's just the worst story I have to tell about Harper Hospital.

I was hysterical. My mother said, "You've got to be kind; you've got to be charitable." My mother is Charity herself. In fact, "Vengeance is mine," says the Lord! And God took care of that guy real well. Because I know that a few years later he had a severely disabled son. And so, he gets to wonder about his own little genes, his little defective genes in bringing about disabled children into the world. But, this was this man's policy. He encouraged people with genetic illnesses to become sterilized.

Recounted Michael about a recent experience:

I tried for our local volunteer fire department. I made it as far as the physical. The doctor walked in the door and she notices the bumps I have on my arms and immediately it is, "Oh, geez, you have von Recklinghausen, huh?" By her attitude, it was almost as though the physical was over. It was as though she had already had it cast in her mind that I had von Recklinghausen and she did not think I should be a fireman. That was basically the end of the physical.

I think the thing that upset me about it the most was that I had already gone through my EMT [Emergency Medical Training] certification, so I am aware of what you might call "bedside manner." I am aware of how you are supposed to deal with people, conduct yourself. And this doctor was to me, very, very unprofessional. Her attitude was almost like she wanted to pull the garlic out of her skirt and hold it up to my face, like, "Oh, you freak, get away from me." [Garlic was used as a medieval protection against witchcraft.] If there was anything at the time I could have done about it, any agency I could have reported her to, I would have. But then it would have boiled down to her word against mine and it would have come down to me being upset because I didn't get my job as a fire fighter.

Misinformation

Many subjects recounted stories of actual misinformation they were given about their condition. Victor bitterly recalled a doctor telling his parents when he was eight years old that he could never play sports. He felt deprived during all of his school years. In his early twenties he was told by another doctor that this advice was not accurate, and that he could have safely participated in sports. The far-reaching implications of medical advice are reflected in this man's discussion of his determination to have children despite the dangers of passing on NF1, which was a serious condition in his mother and siblings.

I think having a kid was kind of like a way to get back for not being able to play football or other sports, not being allowed to go out for sports. It was like I have been robbed of so much because of this skin disease that I want to make up for it. And if I have a kid who has it, I'm going to say, "Let's play ball." I mean, I'm going to figure out some way he can play ball.

And Rachel:

It's weird because my parents were told, "This is a very rare disease and we never see anybody with it and nobody knows about NF. This is a mystery." When, in fact, that's a bunch of bullshit. It's one of the most, I hate to use the word popular, but more continuing birth defects in America. And the bullshit that my parents were fed by doctors who didn't know anything! It's pretty devastating and it's pretty hurtful when you think about it.

Actual stories of bad clinical treatment were much rarer. These situations were recounted by persons with serious early conditions that were discounted or misdiagnosed. Rachel continues:

My NF was discovered when I was eight. In bathing me, my dad found this little lump on my spine the size of a plum. And in a week, it was the size of an apple. So, in other words, the curvature of the spine was starting. And it rapidly got worse and worse. My mother took me to Harper Hospital. And they told her that there was nothing wrong with me. It was all in her imagination.

But what did they say about the back?

They told her there was nothing wrong with me. Everything was in her imagination. They took x-rays. I was in the hospital for a week. And they said there was nothing wrong with me. This was the scoliosis. And they said there was no scoliosis.

There was a doctor who had helped my brother years before at another hospital. We went to see her and she got the x-rays from Harper Hospital. I can remember this big medical conference. All these doctors were sent in to confer. I remember standing up on this table and all these doctors going, "Oooh, look at this; look at this." They made the diagnosis of the NF and they made the diagnosis of the scoliosis. And I was in Barfield Hospital within a week for surgery. The surgeon was great and kind and sweet. I had a series of surgeries from age eight to about seventeen. They kept telling my parents, "We can't address the NF. We can only address the aftermath and do correctional procedures."

And there was a legal ramification. My parents then decided to sue Harper Hospital. And to avoid legal problems they said they would pay for my medical treatment elsewhere. They would pay my hospital bills and surgeon's bills until I was twenty-five, if we chose not to sue. And, there was this wonderful institution then in California called Crippled Children's Services. They paid for the rest of the medical bills. And all my medical workup was done through Barfield Hospital. It was a payoff not to sue. We stayed with the Harper Hospital program, but till I was twenty-five I never saw them for anything about the NF. Now I see a neurologist and an internist at another Harper, who treat me with dignity and respect.

Many persons commented on their lack of timely diagnosis, but the fact that few persons report actual inappropriate treatment in the face of generally poor knowledge or understanding of NF1 by doctors, is in good part because the most severe or serious symptoms of NF1 are relatively rare. Thus most persons who see doctors are not presenting highly at-risk situations.

Several patients reported seeing doctors who use nontraditional modes of treatment or chiropractors. Sarah told me:

I see a woman chiropractor. And she seems to understand quite a bit about what goes on with NF. She sees it as a system disease and not as a condition of tumors, whereas most of the doctors I've seen, they see the tumors aspect and that's all they see. So I found that to be very intriguing. It seems to me most of the really involved help I've had has come from so-called "alternative medicine." Like chiropractors and herbalists, and people like that. And all those people have seen it as a system malfunction disease. She knows I don't have much money, she feels like I'd really benefit from it, so she's charging me a very nominal fee, ten dollars a month and I see her three times a week.

MEDICAL MANAGEMENT STYLES

Subjects had settled into or actively developed a broad array of styles to deal with their medical management. These styles reflect their basic personalities, their parents' patterns of medical management, the nature and severity of their symptoms, and the type of medical resources available to them. The most common pattern of managing the condition was to go in just when there were problems. An almost equal number went for regular or annual check-ups with a general practitioner or internist and then consulted specialists when referred. Although some persons who follow these patterns were very knowledgeable about their condition and kept close watch on their symptoms, in many others a general passivity and sometimes fatalism was apparent. There was often slippage around specific problems, in good part because many doctors do not spontaneously explain medical issues to patients or justify their (doctors') behavior around the patients' care. To complicate this situation, patients often do not ask for sufficient information to allow their understanding, nor do they complain about their treatment or lack of treatment when they are not satisfied.

The vast array of possible symptoms and grades of severity of NF1 may pose significant barriers of confusion to many persons with little education and understanding of complex medical issues. Even persons with considerable education and sophistication encounter difficulties. For example, Nathan describes a serious condition requiring many specialists:

I first saw a dermatologist and I have a general practitioner. He referred me out to various doctors for my problems. I've seen a neurologist, a neurosurgeon, a plastic surgeon. He has done my surgeries at the hospital there.

A plastic surgeon for your tumors?

Well, basically I was having these surgeries, before the cancer [a cancerous tumor in the neck] was diagnosed, I was referred to a plastic surgeon because they knew that ongoingly I would need surgery on and off to remove a tumor. And they thought a plastic surgeon would be good to minimize the scarring. And he brought in some other specialists when he did the tumor in my neck. He brought in a neurologist and a neurosurgeon and had other people there as well to assist, since it was a little bit out of his field. And my basic care doctor now is an oncologist, who is taking care of my cancer treatment and other things. And doing side referrals for me when I need to—like I saw an audiologist, an audiology doctor, about a week or so ago about my hearing, and was taken care of by him. And he's going to be dialoging with my oncology doctor as to what they should or shouldn't do or if anything can be done. So it's quite a hodgepodge of doctors. I kept it all down in writing so I can tell who's who. Plus I'm also seeing, every three months or so now, I'm seeing my radiologist. But he is over at Children's Hospital; they specialize in radiology there. That's where Brandon seems to refer a lot of their cancer patients for radiology treatment. They have a very good system at Children's for that.

In general, how have you felt about your treatment?

I like the care very well. The cancer care, I think, is excellent. The staff is absolutely wonderful. And the doctors there are good. Things are explained. And they treat you like you're intelligent, and with dignity.

I'm also very assertive, to an extent. I was raised in a medical family. I worked for doctors for several years. So I don't hold the medical profession in any state of awe. I know they're human and they can make mistakes. And for the best care, you have to take responsibility yourself too. Like when I go to the doctors I always make sure I have a list of all the problems I'm having, or concerns, and all the questions. I write everything down to make sure I don't miss anything. And so far I've never had any problems with any doctors with that. They seem a little impressed, and they like it because they know I'm willing to take responsibility, and they know when I tell them something, this is it. I'm not holding something back or I'm just not forgetting something. Sometimes just forgetting one little thing can be a problem. I could have not mentioned that tumor and I could have even had worse problems with it.

Nathan, despite his own vigilance and in his perception, good health care, died two months after our interview from an undetected massive brain tumor. He had described the painful cranial symptoms he was having for several months to his doctors and his death occurred four days after a physical examination, but no diagnosis was made until after his death.

Spanning a range of severities, many persons have normalized their lives and try to see doctors as little as possible. Said Michael, who consistently downplays his NF, although he had serious leg surgery early in his life:

My doctor has advised me that I should watch them and see if the tumors increase in size or they get tender or if a tender one gets more tender, and if so, I should go in and see him. But, if there are no changes, not to worry.

Do you ever see any specialists?

No. Lumps and bumps don't seem to bother me. They have been a part of my life for as long as I can remember, so you roll with the punches. Other than having some minor disabilities, coordination problems, to me it's just a part of life. I can't imagine living life another way. It is the way I've been all along so I don't worry about it.

Two persons who have experienced severe lifelong problems requiring extensive surgeries displayed aggressive management styles in their choosing of doctors and their ongoing relationships with them. Both feel that in most cases they have gotten excellent care because of their approaches. Said Sharon, a very seriously affected person whose attitudes and achievements will be discussed in the Conclusion:

I don't believe in just going in for every little thing. And these doctors have this attitude that you don't just take it out because it's there, but that you take it out if it's causing you a problem. But it's not just something that you go and do all the time. And I believe that too. I don't just run in for every little surgery. I've got better things to do with my life. I just go in like anyone else does for regular checkups with my internist. I'm a firm believer that you can't go looking for problems. You go in for a physical just like anyone else going in for a physical and if you are not having any problems, why go to see a neurologist? I don't. Particularly once you are an adult. The old adage applies here: if it is not broken, don't fix it. I think that a lot of people with NF overreact.

I learned from my parents early on in the Midwest that you seek out the best doctors, the best person you can find. I just knew from my father that when something happened to us you just went to the university hospital wherever you were. This was even before I was diagnosed with NF. Now that I'm here, I know that you go to one of the university hospitals and go for the best. People have to learn that they need to take some of the responsibility for their own treatment and care. There are a lot of caring health care professionals out there; we just have to seek them out. My father taught me that, and I really think that doing things like that is learned behavior.

I believe another reason I am so pleased with my medical care is that I do not have unrealistic expectations. That doctor cannot cure my NF. He can help me with whatever problem it is that I am having, but he cannot cure it. He cannot necessarily make it better. Maybe that is why there is a lot of dissatisfaction. Like that woman in the group with her son, Ralph, I mean, how many times does the orthopedic man have to tell her he has done all he can? Now, to some people that would come across as being insensitive. I am sure that sometimes doctors are insensitive. I haven't heard doctors say, "How is your mental health?" I haven't heard that. But that is not their forte. If I am having a problem with my mental state, then I should call a psychiatrist. I mean, I don't go to my gynecologist with that. If I am having a problem there, by the same reasoning, I am not going to call a psychiatrist and say, "Excuse me, I think I'm pregnant."

And I think my positive attitude does help. If you're not obnoxious I think you're going to get good treatment. And I think you're responsible for making sure that you do get good treatment. Like the bad experience I had with the radiation department at Walker Hospital. I let my surgeon know that I wasn't happy and he made sure that that's not where I had my treatments.

I think it also has helped that my sisters and sometimes my brothers-in-law come with me to see the doctor, and they ask a lot of questions too, and are active like I am.

Rudy, a very forceful man who has seen many specialists across the country characterizes his style in dealing with doctors as "aggressive":

I guess I've developed a protective stance. I've spent a lot of time dealing with doctors and all that. I get sort of defensive, especially when I see a doctor. It's not like I go on the defensive; I go on the attack. I don't let doctors get the upper hand with me. I mean, I've surprised some doctors being so—I shouldn't say aggressive—but I guess that's the only way to say it. Like this one famous doctor on the east coast, he came in with five or six of his residents. I knew who the man was. I said, "Hi, how are you? My name is so and so and I know you are Dr. so and so." He sort of took a step back. Most patients don't do that. Especially most patients who've just had a spinal tap. But that's my way. I am aggressive.

You think that developed from your medical history?

I think that's just part of protection. You know, this little kid seen all these doctors. When you're really little you get scared. Especially when they poke and probe and they're not sure what they are going to do. I think I've learned that you never let the physician get the upper hand. A lot of people don't have enough scientific background to be able to do that. I listen to the doctors, you know, from the clinical side; if I heard anything, I'd always try to categorize it. And a lot of people won't do that. It just has to do with medicine. They don't want to hear about it. They just figure the doctor is all-knowing, "Go in there, okay, I'm sick, treat me." Another thing is there's sometimes you ended up trusting a doctor; he says he wants to do that, fine. And I make opinions of doctors very quickly.

What would make for a good favorable opinion? What do you look for?

Each case is different because everybody is different. It's like I work with the public and I have some sensitive interactions and I have to assess each person. I think I've dealt with physicians the same way. Or I trust him because I liked him. There are different manners. There are some that are real professional and come in dignified, and others come in bouncing around or whatever. It's just a feeling I get from them.

The value of others accompanying patients on doctor's visits was brought up by several persons. Lee related that her husband would go with her to the doctor and was very assertive in his manner: "If the doctor would tell us he didn't know something, my husband would tell him, 'Well, if you don't, then find out because we want to know!' He won't stop until he gets an answer. And we're both that way."

Norita described her strategies to get through to hard-to-reach doctors by telephone:

How do you get through to doctors at Harper Hospital?

I leave messages for a week.

And then they'll call you back?

And then they call me back. I call them from nine o'clock on. I say, "I want to speak to Dr. Apperson." I give them my medical number and my name. Then I call at ten o'clock. Then I call at eleven, at twelve, until they get so fed up with me, they say, "Oh, let the doctor speak to her!"

How did you know to do that?

I just thought about it because they were not returning my calls, so I thought, "I'm going to be a pain in the ass, and they're not going to like it." And I tell the doctor, I say, "If you don't return my calls, it's like getting a crab up your butt."

In summary, subjects reported on a wide variety of medical experiences, attitudes toward medical care and specific doctors, and styles of medical management. In this broad range there was little correlation with severity of condition. The more educated (although not necessarily without learning disabilities) and more purposeful and insistent appeared to ultimately receive the best and most satisfying care as reported in their accounts. Implications for medical personnel will be discussed in the Conclusion.

PSYCHOTHERAPY

Eighteen of the affected adults, or one-third of the total, reported that they had seen a professional psychotherapist or attended group therapy led by a professional. Thirteen of these were women and five were men (four of these five men were among the most seriously affected in the sample). Nine of the total eighteen had had multiple psychotherapeutic experiences and reported a mixture of positive and negative ones. Ten reported at least one positive experience; three reported totally positive experiences and three totally negative. Six persons had been in group therapy. Three had attended such groups for specific health concerns and found them useful. Two of the three subjects who reported continual satisfaction with therapists were sophisticated, educated persons with steady employment who could afford private psychotherapy, and who could make the most intelligent choice of the appropriate therapist for their problems and also utilize the therapeutic experience in a productive fashion. The majority of persons who were currently seeing or had recently seen therapists had these services available through their HMOs or county mental health services. Only one of the five persons whose therapy was provided through their HMO health plan was even partially satisfied with the services. Of the six persons who had consulted county mental health services, five were at least partially satisfied with their therapy.

Subjects clearly articulated to me the kinds of problems they felt they had—some NF1-related and some not—and the nature of the help they felt they needed. More frequently than not, when they went to free or low-cost therapy clinics their needs were not respected and they were often mismatched with the therapists they saw. Those subjects who could afford to pay for private therapy were much more satisfied with their therapists and the therapeutic process. Subjects were particularly negative and critical of therapists who refused to recognize or who minimized their psychological or physical pain.

In most cases subjects spent much of their therapy time talking about NF1-related symptoms or consequent problems. However in many other cases NF1-related problems were only peripherally discussed or not at all. Subjects' accounts of their psychotherapy experiences reflect a panoply of life problems apart from those directly or indirectly caused by NF1. This emphasizes the fact that many persons have a host of problems unrelated to NF1 in their lives and their NF1 condition must be seen within the context of the total life gestalt. These contextual problems may be exacerbated by the NF1 or the NF1 may be exacerbated by the contextual problems.

15

Impact

The severe impact of NF1 on the lives of many subjects was apparent throughout the interviews more often in the many ways it pervaded our far-ranging discussions than in direct answers to my questions about it. For example, when I asked Sarah, "Do you have any hobbies or special things that you like to do?" She replied, "I never could develop any hobbies. My task was just survival. Just staying alive was so important to me." And Isabelle, now a quadriplegic:

NF is such a horrible disease! I personally think it's the worse disease a person can have. I don't think cancer or multiple sclerosis or all those things that whoever up there decides to punish you with and can give you are as bad. I don't think there's anything worse than neurofibroma. It's so insidious, it either works on the inside and makes a cripple out of you or it makes you grotesque and ugly. I can't think of anything worse.

And Chuck, surveying his career of surgeries:

I've made a lot of compromises in my life. I compromised about my colostomy and I've compromised about all my surgeries, and everything that my body is doing to me. My mom calls me her hero because I survive and I keep on picking myself up and going on. One of my friends says it's a genetic thing, Jews are taught to be survivors.

In surveying the impact of NF1 on the persons described in this study, we must recognize the distinction between actual physical or debilitating features of NF1 such as external or internal tumors, pain, or mobility or cognitive limitations that subjects may experience, and the societal responses to these manifestations. Social stigma and rejection appear to extract a far more frequent psychological and social price on subjects than do physical symptoms. Yet, disentangling these two dimensions may be difficult indeed, and the impact of NF1 on the lives of individuals and families can be but imperfectly measured in objective terms. Neither severity nor visibility can be considered objective measures for assessing impact. Many persons who appear to be lightly affected relative to others in the sample feel marked by their condition every day of their lives. Likewise others quite visibly or severely affected by clinical standards have stated that they feel their lives would have been little different without the NF1. Corroborating the difficulty in objectifying the impact of NF1 on the lives of affected persons is the finding of Benjamin et al. (1993) that the majority of NF1 patients in their study judged their conditions to be more serious than clinicians had judged them to be.

Individuals often reacted quite differently in their responses to symptoms, thus mediating the impact of NF1 on their lives. For example, many persons with NF1 have poor coordination. Male subjects frequently described their embarrassment at failure in sports activities. They often withdrew from activities requiring physical prowess. Their problems typically were not known at the time to be related to their NF1. Michael's account describes his own stubborn endurance and its cost to his body, a situation that would have been precluded for many other men because of their probable withdrawal from these activities. Said Michael:

> I was very active when I was a child and I have numerous skeletal problems associated with the neurofibromatosis. The coordination problems contributed to the fact that I have skeletal injuries. I raced motorcycles. In reality, I think I spent more time healing than I actually did racing.

> *How is that related to your NF?*

> I think the accidents were because of the lack of coordination. I have broken fingers, and a knee that had surgery on it in high school. I have ankles that are kind of like rubber from, again, just lack of coordination.I have what I jokingly call "radar." If there is something to trip over, my feet will find it. I always thought I had "radar feet" until at one of the [support group] meetings it came out that one of the big problems that people with NF have is the coordination problem. During the ride home, my wife said, "No wonder you're always falling down. I thought you were just clumsy. Now I see there's a reason you're always falling down."

NF1 must be seen as one factor within a context of many others, some of which are the age at the time of interviewing, gender, and personality of the individual; the presence of a family and/or life partner who accepts or does not accept their condition; attitudes of parents; if the individual has first- or second-generation NF1; the presence of learning disabilities; and the utilization of external social supports such as NF support groups.

As one example of the impact of age, as noted in the chapter on marriage, the oldest women in the sample, although quite visibly affected, have not been as obviously bothered by their condition as many of the younger women. They have had long and stable marriages with husbands who have accepted their NF1 as an unremarkable part of their physical persons. Younger persons today, both men and women, who are more influenced by the media and the glaring cosmetic prescriptions for beauty portrayed there, are more aware of their differences, and even the presence of a loving, accepting partner may not deaden their pain. In fact, they may be concerned that a spouse would leave them and they would be unable to find another who could tolerate their appearance or medical problems.

DIMENSIONS OF LIFE IMPACTED BY NF1

The broad range of responses of affected adults about their perceptions of the impact of their NF1 reflected the myriad dimensions of life that they felt had been affected or actually determined. The most frequent responses dealt with societally created problems around appearance and self-image; disenfranchisement from normal expectations for sex, dating, and having children; or limitations on their economic and educational aspirations. Fewer described the daily realities of living with pain or paralysis. Some gave global answers that covered many aspects of their lives. Said Hal:

Well, I think it's definitely limited my job opportunities especially now with my leg. You know, I really can't do anything physical. And socially I have to wait until I find someone who I'm compatible with and doesn't want their own biological kids. Maybe adoption, but even that is iffy, because at any time maybe one of these might go malignant. So it's just a lot of things to really think about.

And Sarah:

For me the socioeconomic factors are that I got ripped off of my opportunities for education just in the circumstances of having repetitive surgeries during that time in a woman's life when she is supposed to be accepted for what she looks like. There is me with a scarred face. I have never been acceptable in that way. It has kept me at a place where I am not able to get an education. Now with a kid it will take me ten years to get through a school program.

Obviously, what I'm doing isn't working. It is just not working. But it is the only thing that I could come up with. If I had access to money it would be totally different. But it is access to money that I cannot get. I honestly believe that at the root of all of this is the NF. It is my condition. I just can't seem to access any of the good stuff. I am pretty much at a point where I feel like throwing in the towel. I am going to spend the next ten years getting a two year degree, and won't be able to use it in the end, anyway. And I will have a child growing up. Also when you work nine hours a day and when you go to school for six hours there is not any time left.

I feel like a rat that has been painted into a corner. When you have a rat that has been cornered, that is when they jump at you. If you chase them, they scurry and scurry, but if they are backed into a corner and there is nowhere to go, they will then attack.

Many adults talked about the impact of NF1 continually as they related various experiences of their lives and discussed their current situations. Some of the complexities of impact are apparent in the following comments. Said Rachel:

You always live on the edge. NF puts you on the edge and leads you to some kind of marginal life. On one level it is either emotionally marginal or physically marginal and economically marginal, as well. I am used to living on the edge. Sometimes I just wish I had the energy to live out that artistic life on the edge. I should be doing something with all these experiences. Maybe if I had more energy at the end of the day I could paint or I could write or I could just do a lot more. I feel it surging inside of me at times. I am finding my way. I know that sounds like a trite statement. Sometimes people say, "How are you?" and I answer, "I am finding my way."

And Rosa:

It's really hard to think of my life being without NF because of the fact that it's been such a big part of my life because of my going to all the doctors, having surgery. Would I be as driven as I am today to try and just do everything that I can? Would I have been a different child, if I hadn't had NF? One of the reasons I was given up for adoption by my natural mother was that she was by herself and she knew I had the disease, and she didn't know if she could take care of me. If I didn't have NF, would my mother have given me up for adoption? And I was in two foster homes prior to my adoptive parents' house. Those foster homes couldn't handle the fact that I had NF because they didn't feel that they could take care of me. So if I hadn't had NF, would I have stayed with one of those families? So you know, I probably would have been this normal little kid running around doing everything everybody else does.

The interrelatedness of the presence of NF1 and its symptoms with a multitude of lifestyle factors could be illustrated by the cases of several women in the sample who had exceedingly poor self-images as young adults and, by their accounts, desperately married the only men who courted them. These men proved to be dysfunctional husbands and fathers, and also poor economic providers, resulting in marginal economic situations. These women showed up poorly in invidious family economic comparisons and were looked down on by their siblings. They felt ostracized by their families of orientation.

Physical Attractiveness

Problems of self-image and physical attractiveness were mentioned by the most persons when talking about the effects of NF1 on their lives. Said Annie:

It has affected my self-esteem. And I think self-esteem affects all aspects of your life. Whether it be advancing yourself in your job or your education. You know, I would never ever enter a beauty pageant. Not that that's a necessary thing in life, but do you know what I'm saying? I would never ever do something like that. I never liked going to bars or the "in" places to meet men, because I thought, "Well, who is going to be attracted to me?" So there are certain things I held back and I didn't do because of my image of my NF.

Said Ronald:

What my NF has contributed to within the last four or five years is my self-esteem. Since I've started using a cane, I still have a high regard for myself as a human being, but I feel very inhibited for going out and meeting women and trying to establish a relationship.

Emotional Impact

Several women observed that their experience in dating and developing intimate relationships was greatly retarded. They considered that the resultant stultifying of their emotional and social sophistication was a by-product of their NF1 and has caused them severe problems in their adult life. Said Norita, "It has been a big hit for me emotionally. I have not had time to grow up, to develop, because of being protected by my mother because of what I had. She prevented me from getting out into the world."

Most of those persons whose NF1 was visible in childhood talked about its negative influence on their early life and developing personalities. Often the NF1 compounded or exacerbated other physical or family problems. For example, said Norita:

I was very depressed when the doctor told me about my NF. A lot of things happened during that time. I was raped. I tried to commit suicide. From September to December I found out I had this and that I wasn't going to get better and that it might even get worse. At that point I thought, "This is what I am going to get; this is what I am going to look like." I didn't want to look like that. And then, a few days before Thanksgiving, my mother's best friend's son raped me and after that I just lost the will to live. I was very depressed being in this country, having such a hard time. And I thought, "This is what I get for coming to this country. God is punishing me for betraying my people and not staying there." That's how I thought at that time. I didn't understand about the genes and all that.

Economic Impact

Economic implications were mentioned frequently. Many persons spoke bitterly of the learning disabilities that they feel closed off major economic possibilities for them. Said Robbie:

I did lose some jobs because of my dyslexia. I was let go from some positions because I made some clerical mistakes. One time it was for a lawyer on a case. I got things all mixed up. He didn't tell me this; I found out second hand because I wasn't in the office the day it was discovered. But I flubbed up. So I lost that. I've lost about seven jobs because of either not being able to learn something fast enough or from making a major mistake.

The necessity for time off for surgeries impacted negatively on many persons' work careers. For example, Sarah commented, "I've never been in a situation where I could build any kind of safety net. I've had quite a few surgeries, and it's not like that sort of thing is going to affect your life or your pocketbook on a short term basis."

Pain and Severity

About one in ten affected adults in the sample described constant pain or specific physiological sensations or conditions that often limit their activities or dictate their lives. This account in my field notes is an example:

Rachel and I were in a shop looking at some Frida Kahlo [Mexican painter] paintings reproduced on cards, and there was one nude painting of Kahlo which portrayed her spinal column like a cracked Greek column, with nails in all parts of her body. Rachel said, "Oh I had this painting hanging over my bed when I was a teenager. I thought this was me. Everything about it was me. The pain, essentially the pain, and the broken way her body was." [Rachel related her own scoliosis and many surgeries to the situation of Kahlo who had been seriously injured in a streetcar wreck in her teenage years and also suffered through many surgeries and much pain. Kahlo's image became Rachel's metaphor for her own pain.]

And Lou, who lived with a severe scoliosis, said, "The NF is with me all the time because I am in constant pain. Since I've gotten older, I think there has been a change in my back and I have mostly pain every single day. I'd just like to get up and not have any pain one day." And Harry, who often talked about his continual back pain:

I've been taking this Tylenol® with codeine for a long time. I'm not addicted; I'm past the point of being addicted. I mean, that's way back yonder by now. The Tylenol doesn't kill the pain; it just makes it tolerable. You know, there's some nights I pace the floor all night. Now I'm just to the point that the pain's getting worse and it's getting harder and harder to deal with it.

Chuck discussed the practical problems of daily life and relationships resulting from surgeries from his NF1 tumors:

I was very, very devastated by the surgery. After many years I still don't like dealing with the ostomy. It's even hard for me to even say the word "ostomy." It's kind of a difficult thing to discuss. I don't like it. I see it as a very ugly part of my body, and it's always going to be there. I can't leave my house in the morning without the irrigations every day. If I want to go anywhere, I have to be up an hour and a half before finally leaving the house. Every day I have to be at work at the office at seven-thirty, so I'm up at five-thirty.

I can't go camping, because how do I go camping when there are no bathroom facilities for me to use? Any long-distance trips I plan I have to make sure I have all my equipment with me. I have to bring backups and spares, so it's actually a major part of my life.

I think my colostomy is definitely a handicap. I do know that there are certain places where I can't go to the bathroom; there are certain places where I cannot do what I have to do every morning. I know like when I stay with a girl I have to bring my overnight kit, and bring all my stuff there and have to set up there. Sometimes a girlfriend's bathroom is too small and might keep us from being intimate because it would have been a problem because the bathroom was too small for me to get into to set myself up that way. So I definitely see it as a handicap. I can't just pick up and go somewhere; I always have to make sure my equipment is with me if I'm going to be away overnight. As far as the NF goes, I see the NF as being the direct cause of the ostomy. So I see that as causing my handicap. They say that you learn to adjust and adapt to it, and the best I've ever done was learn to put up with it. And that's a direct result of the tumors so I get angrier. If I blame the disease for anything, I blame it for that.

Issues of life and death take on immediate importance for severely affected persons. For example, Chuck:

When I was getting involved with my girlfriend I told her, "I can't really make a commitment to you. I don't know how long I've got, and for me, I really want to be in a committed relationship. I want to be in a relationship where thirty years from now I'm going to be waking up next to the same person, but I'm also aware that I may not be here thirty years from now, and so I have problems becoming committed to somebody because of it. I can't commit to you; you've got your life; I may be dead in ten years." And her attitude was, "Well, I'll take you for as long as I can get you." That was the attitude, and it was a nice attitude.

And Robbie:

They did an MRI scan and they found quite a large tumor just a hair's breadth from my seventh vertebrae. My case went before the ethics board because the issue was if the surgery was not successful there would be damage to the seventh vertebrae, which would mean I would have been paralyzed from the neck down and on a resuscitator. And the decision I had to make was would I want to be resuscitated, brought out of the surgery, if there was that damage? And I decided, "No, I would not." And the ethics board agreed with me. So I went into surgery knowing that if it wasn't successful I would not be waking up. But I did wake up, wiggled my toes and fingers and I didn't see any breathing equipment around, so I figured, "Oh, the surgery was a success."

Isabelle, now a quadriplegic, voiced her despondency as she described her active former life:

It's made me want to die. I never was a person that wanted to die. I wanted to live, to be like my father and mother. My mother was remarkable; she was eighty-six, and had a beautiful figure and she dyed her hair black and she would walk all around. We were all walkers in my family, which is ironic. That's what I did for a hobby, walked. My mother and I used to walk for hours. And I never thought about wanting to die. I wanted to see my kids grow up; I wanted to see what was going to happen in the world. The world is so exciting with everything that's going on. But now I have no reason to wake up in the morning. I wake up and I'm either going to have an enema or a shower and then I'm going to lie here and watch TV. I've become hooked on soap operas which I thought would never happen to me. I just don't see any point in living; I can't look forward to anything.

Four persons, three women and one man, disclosed that they had made unsuccessful suicide attempts in moments of desperation related to unending painful surgeries, paralysis, or social consequences of their condition.

Effects on Personality

Several persons commented that their condition had made them more sensitive, understanding individuals or in other ways had positively affected their personalities. Said Robbie:

I do think that I am more sensitive to other people than I might have been had I not had NF. I am not a judgmental person. I don't look at people and say, "Oooh." I don't know if I would or would not be this way if I had not had NF. I think I am a good person inside. I don't think that I judge people on what they look like, that this is not what makes a person a person. You could be the most beautiful person in this world and be the cruelest, ugliest person that ever lived to other people and this would take away from your inner beauty.

And Lou:

In my opinion, it did make me a stronger person. And when I was younger if I did see another person that had a disability or something like that, it made me not stare or make fun of them, because I know how it is to be made fun of or stared at. If you have NF, you just have to live day to day. Just take it in stride as much as you can.

Sometimes I kind of make jokes about it, but I do think the NF made me stronger. I guess I take it in stride. I think if my sister had my problem, she would be in the nut house. She worries over dumb little stupid things like, "Do you think I should eat this before I eat that?" She worries about herself so much. I just don't think she could have handled what I went through. Because they have worked on me [many surgeries] ever since I was thirteen years old, it just made me see things in another light. People say, "Boy, with what you've been through and you crack jokes!" I never did see a therapist about it or anything like that.

AWARENESS OF THE CONDITION

One indicator of impact is the level of consciousness of the NF1 condition. Responses to my questions about consciousness ranged from those given by persons who are never free from the special concerns of NF1, through those who think about it only when they look in the mirror or are aware of the stares or comments of others, to those who very rarely think about it. The presence of specific problems such as tumors that the individual considers unsightly or bothersome or issues of surgery may throw the condition into a momentary spotlight. The consciousness of NF1 tends to be triggered by subjects' daily viewing of visible tumors, or by others staring at them, or by continual pain or other symptoms. Typically more women stated that they think about their NF1 daily. Rachel talked about the personal implications of her consciousness:

NF's been like my shadow, so this makes me very conscious of my NF. It is that part of me that I can never lose. A lot of people live in denial. I think, once you get to a point of consciousness, you become in fact, empowered. The outside forces of the world may try prejudice against you, they may try to manipulate you, they may try to discriminate against you. But they can't once you're conscious about it, because you are powerful and you can say "no." It's like learning to empower children against abuse. You just let them know that they can actually bring forces in the world to their beck and call. My NF is my shadow. And one of the powerful memories I have of my first awareness of NF was that my shadow changed. You know, playing on the playground, as my back started to curve [with scoliosis], as the curvature became more and more dramatic, I saw the shadow on the playground change and how terrible that was. That's a really vivid memory, feeling unable to force myself to stand up, to make it right. So, the NF is in some way a powerful tool that keeps me conscious.

Several men with serious internal tumors talked about the necessity for daily vigilance concerning the possibility of new and dangerous symptoms developing. Their health concerns are tied in with economic ones about health coverage and issues of missing work and threatening their employment. Said Randy:

The major impact on me is having to keep a constant watch on my health, having to know that if I get a stomach ache, if it lasts more than two days, is it the flu? Is it problems with my intestines? If it's there a week then am I having more problems? Do I have to go out and have scans done? If I feel a lump somewhere, is it just a bruise or is it a hydrocele? Do I have to keep a watch on every single lump in my body? It's like, "Yeah, we're going to have to remove that piece of tumor." "Okay, how long am I going to be out, a week? Is it going to be two weeks? Is it going to be six months? How much money do I have in my savings? Can I afford to live on disability for five months or five weeks?"

Others described matter-of-fact attitudes toward their intermittent awareness. Said Clarise:

I think about it like once every two or three weeks. Usually the only time it enters my brain during the day is if someone looks at me funny. At those times, I may get a little self-conscious about it. It is only if I find someone staring at me. It never really obsesses me.

About one-fifth of the adult subjects stated that they consciously do not let their NF1 dictate or severely color their lives. For example, stated Theresa:

I don't dwell on it. I have it. There's nothing I can do to make it go away. I always try to live by the philosophy that you accentuate the positive. It's only when someone says something, and then inside of myself, I may feel self-conscious. But I know that my husband loves me for me. When I go to buy clothes, I'll buy the long sleeves. I have a lot of women friends. I get along fine with the men I work with. I'm self-conscious, yes. But I don't dwell on it.

I used to be shy in my earlier years but I have become more assertive, because you find out that it doesn't make you as a person; it doesn't mean that you're going to be left on your job. I do very well. I interface with senior vice-presidents. I interface with secretaries and all categories of persons. The NF is not going to stop me from having good friends, or interfacing with people. It's only if you let it. I used to be very shy, very quiet, very held back, but now I am just going to have a good time.

It should be noted that the above statement was made by a woman whose NF1 symptoms are as fully noticeable as some of those who state they think about their condition daily or even continually. This underlines the subjective factors that may determine an affected individual's response to her or his physical condition. In some cases this may be strong family support, professional accomplishment, or a developed "attitude" that is related to a positive self-image.

Several persons stated that they believe neither they nor others should blame their NF1 for all the problems in their lives. Said Sharon, an introspective woman who is both visibly and severely affected:

I think it is too easy to blame NF for your own troubles. We all have to take a certain responsibility for our lives. I think now, that certainly my life is different having had this, like people who are blind would be different had they been able to see and like people who are obese would have been different had they not been obese. We all have to deal with the temple that we have been given and we live in a very "perfect" society. I mean, the Diet Pepsi commercials feature all these anorexic, gorgeous, young, affluent people. And for people with NF, the reason they're being judged is just because of their appearance, not because they have or don't have NF. I mean, there are other people with other afflictions that are also thought to be awful and made fun of. It is not just because it is NF. I have done an awful lot of soul searching lately. The "stop-smoking" program I went to was wonderful because they really make you think, and they teach you to take responsibility for your own life and to be aware that we all have choices in our lives. The mind is a magnet and you can create anything if you focus your mind on it.

I don't know whether my unsuccessful relationships with men have to do with me and have nothing to do with NF. NF is just not my convenient excuse. "Well, he didn't call again and had I not had NF, he would have called again." I mean, maybe I talk too much about myself; maybe I talk too much about my mother. I don't know yet what it is, but I need to look at the fact that if it is not just one or two people, maybe it is something else that I am doing. I don't think I can blame all of my misfortunes on NF. And oftentimes, even if it is NF, you need to say, "I choose to go on and have a productive life. I choose to have control over my own happiness." I can sit around and be miserable and say, "Oh, poor me!" Or, I can keep trying. And I think I want to keep trying. I haven't always felt this way. Maybe I am getting older and this has begun to become important in my life.

And Chuck spoke of surviving several very serious surgeries that have also determined the logistics of his dating and limited his aspirations for marriage and fatherhood:

I don't know if it's actually affected me socially or not. I never really thought about it as being something that is a social deterrent to me. I think it comes back to my dealing with it matter-of-factly; that's the only way I'm able to. I can disassociate it. . . . [Later in the interview] I've always thought my loneliness was because I don't have anyone. I never thought it was because of the NF but since I feel that I may die in ten years because of this disease, and I wonder how can I ask some woman to spend the rest of her life with me when the rest of my life may be ten years, so I do go through that sometimes.

Chuck's symptoms were extremely serious and life-threatening. He recounted problems in beginning and maintaining relationships, some of which were doubtlessly related at least indirectly to his NF1, yet he did not necessarily attribute these social problems to his condition. In the cases of Chuck and many other persons the subjectivity of personal assessments of the impact of NF1 was clearly apparent.

16

Conclusions: Living Alone with Genetic Disorder

Neurofibromatosis 1 is a lonely disorder. The heterogeneity of its presentation—the possibility of many seemingly unconnected and sometimes serious symptoms—may demand individualized idiosyncratic adaptations. Most genetic disorders exhibit a similarity of symptoms among individuals in the same family, if not with all others with the condition. However, the diversity of symptoms of NF1, even within members of the same family, may serve to make each feel that his or her own condition is uniquely bad, making for barriers in communication between parent and child and between siblings. Some subjects report that their doctors told them that their condition was not serious, thus any children they might have with the disorder would have a likewise mild or moderate case. However, as noted above, in at least six cases children's conditions were much more serious than those of their parents. The distinctness of each case is underlined by these examples. Further, the lack of common expectations discourages not only family communication but may preclude the benefits of social support from NF support groups or other sources.

As noted in Chapters 10 and 13, the uncertainty around NF1 may discourage individuals and families from attending NF support group meetings for fear of seeing others with frightening symptoms they themselves might one day experience. If they do attend meetings, they may find they have little in common with others there. This heterogeneity of symptoms may be very much in evidence when members describe their symptoms and concerns. While some persons may have visible symptoms, others report nonvisible ones, such as skin tumors on clothed parts of the body, internal tumors ranging from those in the cranium to the feet, or learning disabilities and serious problems of coordination. Participants who do not share these specific symptoms may then start to worry, "Could I develop this at that age?" or "Could my child develop this?" Ironically, although designed to assist members, support groups might then provide the staging grounds for more anxiety and feelings of aloneness.

PERSONAL ADAPTATION TO NF1 AND AMERICAN SOCIETY

How have the persons portrayed in this study adapted to their condition and survived in a "beauty"-conscious society where attaining social and financial success may be extremely difficult or even impossible for those with complex and far-reaching health conditions? What are the factors that have entered into their struggles, helping or hindering them? In order to explore these issues I propose an assessment of personal adaptation to NF1 and to the demands of the society in which we live. Personal adaptation is a difficult and tenuous concept to objectively describe or measure. With temerity I propose to assess personal adaptation by applying three criteria: (1) a proactive accepting, if not positive, attitude toward one's condition; (2) development of pragmatic coping abilities; and (3) being able to meet or succeed in normative or common societal life cycle accomplishments in economic and social spheres of life, that is, employment, marriage, and the development of social relationships. I ranked subjects by attitudes and abilities exhibited in (1) and (2) and the degree of achievement of (3). The breakdown was: "*Good*"—twenty-nine; "*Fair*"—fifteen; and "*Poor*"—ten.

I will consider below how the variables of gender, age at diagnosis, presence of NF1 in a parent, socioeconomic status of parents, learning disabilities, visibility, severity, and available social support networks are related to adaptation.

Gender: As a group, women appear to have adapted better than men. Six of the ten poor copers were women and four men, however numerically there were one-third more women than men in the sample overall. Of the fair copers eight were women and seven men, and of the good copers, nineteen were women and ten, men. The men who have done well have tended to come from a favored early environment of strong parental support and/or adequate finances to assist them in continuing in school even when severe learning disorders were present. However as noted in Chapter 9, five men out of the total of twenty-two withdrew as teenagers from the expectations and challenges of social life.

Age at Diagnosis: The literature on chronic disease and disability suggests that an early diagnosis of a lifelong condition may facilitate a more successful acceptance of and adaptation to the condition. I did not find early age at diagnosis necessarily to be a predictive factor for a successful adaptation. In fact, unless the affected child had strongly positive and supportive parents who instilled assertiveness and a strong self-image in the child, those diagnosed in childhood had no better outcomes in relation to their coming to terms with their condition.

One very articulate woman commented on how glad she was to have learned of her condition at eight years old, because this gave her time to learn about and adapt to what would come, even though her parents appear not to have been stalwarts in helping her. Yet, another said that she was glad she did not find out about her NF1 until she was twenty, because she thinks her parents would have responded poorly thus engendering a poor early response from her.

The teenage years also were not a promising period for subjects to learn about their condition. In fact those diagnosed in their early teenage years had among the worst outcomes in terms of later developing adequate coping patterns. The young and older adult years seem to be the best time for individuals to be diagnosed, even though a number of persons described their pain at learning of their condition during pregnancy or childbirth, or at the time of their child's diagnosis. While prior knowledge might have persuaded them not to have children, in terms of their own lives they usually had achieved a normal lifestyle by the time of diagnosis. They had jobs and were married, and sometimes already had other children. Many of these persons were mildly affected, both in visibility and severity, which in part accounts for their late diagnosis. Since their late diagnosis however, four have developed problems of high severity and three of great visibility.

Presence of NF1 in a Parent: The familiarity with NF1 in a child's household was no predictor of a good outcome. In fact, those persons who had a parent who was affected but did not communicate with the child about their shared condition often were racked with fears and uncertainties about their own condition and resentments toward their parent with the condition. Five of the ten poor copers and five of the fifteen fair copers had a parent with the condition. However, those few parents who did have good communication with their children about their shared condition did contribute to good attitudes and coping. In those rare instances where parents talked openly to their children about their conditions, told them what they might expect from NF1, and provided emotional support, even persons with extremely severe or visible conditions have made good adaptations.

Socioeconomic Status of Parents: While the socioeconomic status of parents of good copers ranged from affluent to impoverished, the range was far narrower for the poor copers. Among the poor copers one person was born into an upper-middle-class family and this family was very dysfunctional. The others with only several exceptions came from solid working-class, fairly stable families. Yet these families rarely had the educational background and financial resources to give their children, whether diagnosed early or not, the push and advantages that later would spell out successful school and work experiences for specially challenged individuals. Of the nine minority group persons in the sample, three were in the poor coping category. However, ethnicity appeared to play little role in subjects' responses to NF1. No distinct patterns of behavior were noted in these small subsamples that could be correlated with ethnicity.

Learning Disabilities: Learning disorders profiled as the major symptom that was talked about by those subjects who relayed problems. All ten of the poor copers described learning disabilities that hobbled them throughout their lives. They frequently described miserable school experiences and disappointing work careers in jobs that they could not manage, or that were not interesting or satisfying in terms of content and remuneration. Despite whatever other symptoms may have existed, their poor achievement records and lack of self-confidence appear to have affected them more seriously in terms of school and job achievements. Nine of the fifteen fair copers reported significant learning problems. Of the good copers, at least nine had learning disorders. These persons typically had positive family support and/or sufficient resources to assist their early adaptation.

Visibility: Most of the subjects would be categorized as mildly or moderately visible. However, of the eighteen I classified as highly visible because of numerous obvious tumors or problematic skeletal features, at least one-third have adapted well to their condition, and have positive, proactive approaches to the problems of their lives. Half of these persons displayed very visible symptoms from childhood on. They all had strong proactive parents who early on instilled self-confidence and assertiveness in them as young children. Each received excellent medical care during childhood. Two of the oldest persons in the sample had very visible tumors at the time of my interviews but these had been little apparent until well into their adulthood. These two also came from three or more generation NF1 families in small towns where their condition was known and accepted. Six of the ten poor copers had highly visible conditions, and three others had moderately visible conditions, but their lack of social and economic success in most cases was due to their learning disorders and associated problems rather than visible features.

Severity: Fifteen persons were classified as having very severe conditions. Of those, six persons had made good adaptations. One person's condition was not officially diagnosed until late in life. His learning disabilities were camouflaged throughout his career in private schools and family businesses. The other five had severe and in most cases highly visible conditions. They had early ready family social and emotional support and in all but one case sufficient family economic resources that helped them throughout college. In fact, all of these persons were college graduates. Of the other nine persons in the high-severity category, only two were college graduates and they had had problematic childhoods. Six persons ranked in the highly severe category were classified as poor copers. Seven persons were either chronically depressed or stated they were significantly depressed at the time of interviewing. Six were on disability benefits, three of these related to psychiatric conditions. Ten of the fifteen reported learning disabilities through their lives. The fair or good copers in this high-severity category conquered this challenge through family assistance and a personal drive to get through college.

Social Support Networks: Eight of the ten poor copers reported they had a dearth of current social relationships. They had few friends and the several who attended churches or other social groups stated these were not helpful or satisfying. Four erratically attended NF support group meetings that were held in their area, but the information gleaned there helped only two of these and the others not at all in making them more effective copers or more comfortable with their condition. Perhaps the striking point about this group is that seven of these persons described weak, unhelpful, or even destructive early family relationships. Four of the five persons who had a parent with NF1 reported no communication with their parent that was emotionally or practically helpful. Seven of the fair copers also reported a dearth of relationships.

DISCUSSION

Coming of age in the last half of the twentieth century has posed numerous social and economic challenges for all who have experienced it. And for persons who carry their own special health challenges, such as NF1, the tasks of daily life may be even more daunting. For example, because learning disabilities, more than other visibly apparent features of NF1, have tended to hobble the affected individuals in this study, one might ask, "Well then, what is the difference between these persons and those many others in the mainstream society with learning disabilities but no other special health condition such as NF1? This population is estimated to be perhaps as large as 10 percent of the population of the United States. Why should people with NF1 be any worse off than the others without NF1?" My interviews and observations have convinced me that many affected persons have lived within a debilitating global syndrome of NF1, a mystique constituted by the many varying dimensions of the disorder, often inseparable from the issue of learning disabilities: (1) the knowledge that one lives with a genetic disorder that inhabits and has inhabited every cell of his/her body since birth and will remain until death; (2) an accompanying feeling of shame or stigma attached to the *idea* of genetic disorder; (3) the presence or the possibility of disfiguring physical symptoms that could visibly maim one for life in even the simplest necessary social forays of daily existence; (4) living with uncertainty about the possible progression of the condition, a coexistence that invites anxiety that may cloud all areas of life; and (5) feeling disenfranchised from ordinary choices around reproduction, knowing that there is a 50 percent chance of passing on the condition, and in the case of women, possibly worsening one's own condition.

This study has focused on those aspects of subjects' lives that have been most impacted by their NF1 condition. Even those good copers who reported few social and economic problems that they connect with their NF1 talked about sometimes serious problems with which they have managed to cope effectively. The lives of these persons have been marked but not critically shaped by NF1.

In considering the complex interplay of factors that have come together in subjects' lives, perhaps the most salient feature is that neither severity nor visibility of the NF1 condition can predict with certainty the kind of adaptation that any individual will make. Silenced by a history of failure in many areas of life, depressed by a personal appearance that the daily barrages of the media proclaim to be less than valued in this society, and sometimes barely subsisting on the economic margins of society, many persons are resultantly negative about their bodies, their minds, their past, and their future. However, others who share the same factors that could make for despair have maintained a positive and even upbeat attitude, are demanding and energetic in their quests for medical care and for a satisfying social life. And indeed, their positive approach appears to draw positive responses from employers, doctors, and friends.

A case in point of those who despite numerous health problems maintain a positive determination to normalize their lives is Sharon, a lively and personable woman who early in her college career quit formal schooling, but has made herself highly employable through on-the-job training programs and is now a business analyst for a large software company. Her vitality, enthusiasm, industry, and dedication have made her very attractive to supervisors wherever she has worked. Following a series of surgeries for malignant internal neck and thoracic tumors, she has made her way through numerous rounds of radiation and chemotherapy, continuing to work whenever humanly possible. She has won the admiration and affection of her doctors and received excellent medical attention ("I always search out the best there are."). Throughout her weight and hair losses she has smiled and joked, buying five wigs, and becoming a mainstay of her cancer support group. During our interviews and discussions, which have spanned eight years, Sharon has always emphasized the positive aspects of her life. She has maintained a very attractive, well dressed appearance, a beautifully appointed apartment, and a coterie of doctors who deeply care about her well-being. Said Sharon:

We need to get beyond victimhood. We cannot change what life has dealt us, but what we do with our life is our responsibility. You can make yourself miserable. If you are feeling down and allow yourself to feel that way, you'll stay down. When you are depressed have you ever tried doing something to force yourself out of it, like putting on really upbeat music and maybe dancing around? You start to feel better. Unfortunately, we don't always do that. We sit down and do nothing and we just keep feeling worse and worse. But people have to *want* to feel better. And if somebody doesn't want to feel better, no matter what you do, no matter what kind of song and dance you go through, you're not going to change the way you feel.

During one of her rounds of chemotherapy, Sharon observed:

I can't change the fact that I have NF; I can't change the fact that I'm being treated for cancer; I can't change those things. I can change the way I feel about things. I do have control over the way I live my life. You know, it's much more fun to laugh than it is to cry. Crying ruins your make-up. [Laughing] I just think that it's really important to keep your sense of humor, and be the first one to laugh at yourself.

Michael also frequently emphasized his positive orientation:

Some people at the meetings seem to get a little emotional about it. They're a little different from my view which is, as long as you can live with this disability, there are worse things that can happen to one. NF is not up there with MS and AIDS and all sorts of things that can happen to the body that can put you into a wheelchair for the rest of your life. I can still go camping or I can jump on my bicycle and ride around in the mountains. Sure, I have a disorder; I have something wrong with me, but gosh, it could be a whole lot worse. And I don't care if you don't like my NF. If you don't like my appearance, if you don't like the lumps and bumps, there's the door and you can go out the door! There's a whole world waiting to accept me!

And Randy, who has experienced many surgeries for internal tumors:

What would I tell some kid who is facing surgery? I would tell him, "Emotionalize about it; cry about it; punch a wall or two (just don't poke holes in it, otherwise your parents will get very angry at you). Maybe kick a brick down the block; sit there and mope; feel sorry for yourself. But when you're done doing all of that, figure out what you're going to do when it's over, and do it." That's what I would tell him to do. And you know, I would even tell him, "It's okay for you to sit there and cry; it's okay for you to sit there and complain, 'why the hell is this happening to me?' It's okay for you to sit there and feel sorry for yourself; and if anyone tells you it's not, tell them to go to hell. Because it's okay for you to do that. And it's even okay for you to be depressed about it for six months. But that's it. What's not okay is for you to let it ruin your whole life."

Hell, if I'm not being cut on every two years I think something is wrong. One time I told somebody that I probably have more scars than the Frankenstein monster does. You know, it's a joke, but I do have a lot of scars. I do have my worries, and I do have my depression, and I do have my crying fits about those things when they happen, but they're happening and I can't stop them. When the emotions run those courses I sit down and say, "Okay, now that I've emotionalized it, how do I solve it?"

I figure no matter how shitty life gets, as long as you're alive, it's better than the alternative. And as long as you're alive you can survive anything. As long as you know that you're going to wake up the next day, then that's what you can look forward to.

Harry, a very visibly and severely affected man, also described his positive philosophy for living:

I go out in the public eye a lot. I don't go out there with the feeling that there is anything wrong with me. I think these people who have deformities and have problems, it is the way they come across. If they come across as a positive person, and use their mind, I think anybody can be anything they want to be. Go out and boat! Go out and swim! Go out and play golf! It should be brought into the public. They should live their lives like whatever so-called normal people do, whatever that means. It's not the end. You go on with your life like everybody else.

Attitudes and "Attitude"

As I describe the challenges of NF1, it may be useful to consider how persons with two other physically visible genetically based conditions with which I am familiar, dwarfism and osteogenesis imperfecta type III and type IV (OI), manage the challenges of their lives. This discussion is presented knowing full well that genetic conditions or physical disabilities cannot be *compared* in terms of their effects on individuals. Each person perceives the severity of their condition in relation to the realities of their own life. However it is instructive to have the perspective on how persons with differing conditions have managed their lives and what possibilities have assisted them. Most dwarfs, or little people, told me that before they joined the national organization of Little People of America (LPA), they had denied their dwarfism—even in the face of such constant societal reminders as staring, teasing, or social snubs. After joining LPA and passing successfully through the often difficult ritual of having to confront the realities of their own identity as "dwarf" by being forced to view others with their same body configuration, they experienced a *cognitive restructuring* of the self-image. They were able to experience their lives more happily and securely. Much of their security was brought to them through the social power of LPA. They found a community of persons who shared their same physical features and social experiences. They saw attractive role models who had families, jobs, and homes, and they realized that essentially all of the benefits of life were also available to them and to the dwarf children they might have (Ablon 1984). As mentioned earlier, their optimism is reflected in the growing birthrate of dwarf children who, likewise, will look forward to a bright future for persons of physical difference. The security and confidence that many dwarfs now feel about themselves and their physical condition may be seen in the following statement that appeared in a recent LPA national newsletter concerning a surgical procedure that is able to lengthen the limbs of short-statured persons:

Proponents of limb lengthening tend to view the procedures as a "cure" to dwarfism. To me, it is fairly provocative to even think that dwarfism is a condition that needs a cure. What does this say about us as human beings? While in our youth, we may have questioned why am I so short? But as we grew older, we became less concerned with this question and focused our attention to promoting our abilities while gaining self-confidence and self- esteem as we were able to adapt our lives in a society where many things were out of reach or unobtainable. Many of us, if given a chance, still would not change who we are or how tall we might be. While we all face "challenges" to some degree or another, we are who we are. For a majority of us, our affiliation with LPA has made our lives easier, and unless you were a kid when you joined LPA, we haven't grown an inch. . . .

The proclaimed "functional improvements" from limb lengthening have to be viewed with some skepticism as they generally do not rectify the barriers placed upon us by society's attitudes that people of difference and diversity must conform to the norm. . . .

We focus our energy to make our society more accommodating as a way to provide more opportunities for dwarfs to improve the quality of their lives. LPA has evolved over the years and collectively, our efforts have made life easier for dwarfs, while also building upon our self-esteem and presence in our own communities. (McCulloh 1998:14)

The condition of NF1 poses certain obstacles that dwarfism, for example, achondroplasia, the most common type of dwarfism, does not carry with it. While persons with NF1 typically are of normal or near-normal height and body configuration, thus not so readily recognizable as physically different, persons with achondroplasia ordinarily do not exhibit learning disorders, the feature most disabling in the population of affected persons described here. Further, the parameters of achondroplasia and other types of dwarfism are well known. Individuals and families know the extent of their condition. They do not live with the uncertainty of wondering how far their condition might proceed. However, many little people described to me the loneliness and social insecurities they experienced before gaining a strong social group composed of persons with whom they could relate. Persons with NF1 typically do not feel a bond with others with their condition. The example of dwarfism suggests that support groups for NF1, which purposefully strive to get beyond the features of the condition which work against personal identification with others in the group, could begin to provide a strong basis for then making available varied resources for enhancing self-image and engendering confidence for greater success in social life and employment.

The second population that provides a vivid contrast to NF1 is that of persons with OI type III and type IV. These persons share a connective tissue disorder of poor collagen synthesis. Persons affected have very brittle bones, and experience numerous breaks until the late teens. One hundred breaks of the legs and arms before age sixteen are not unusual. Affected persons typically are quite small—adults often weigh less than seventy pounds and are in power wheelchairs. The physical aspect of these persons is even more readily apparent than are those of most dwarfs. Their lower limbs are often quite short and their bodies may be configured differently. The many adults I have interviewed have experienced frequent hospitalizations, sometimes for many months; years of missing school; and severe limitations on their employment possibilities. The problems of living, like those of persons with NF1, often have been caused by the societally-created barriers of prejudice and the inaccessibility of their environments, not by inherent physical differences. Despite the facts of their lives that might be expected to lead to despondency and fatalism, persons with OI are known by professionals who deal with them to be assertive and cheerful. Indeed, I have found the persons I have interviewed to be extremely independent, most achieving professional and social success. They have what in contemporary parlance is called "attitude." They feel that, "If you don't like it that I weigh fifty-seven pounds and am in this chair, I'm sorry, but *too bad.*"

A multitude of factors appears to have brought persons with OI to this feeling of independence even before joining any support group of the Osteogenesis Imperfecta Foundation. Years of hospital trips and painful surgeries, often having to teach health care professionals how to handle and treat their bodies, and limited activity choices compared to their peers, have brought forth a motivation to achieve the maximum that they can and to overcome barriers of physical fragility and oftentimes negative family situations. While experiencing severe physical problems, this population does not exhibit learning disabilities, which persons with NF1 have often represented to have adversely shaped much of their lives. Persons with OI appear to have come on their own, individually, to the fundamental philosophic and practical orientation of the disability rights movement. *Disability is rooted in the environment, not in a physical difference or deficiency of an individual.* If persons with NF1 could come to this awareness, the onus of the burden of NF1 for the individual could be significantly lightened in many cases.

How can persons with NF1 proceed along this positive and proactive path? Years of reinforced failure make this a significant challenge indeed. However, NF organizations and NF clinics have the resources and networks for outreach to develop support groups specifically for adults designed to transcend the diversity of symptoms and lifestyles and to emphasize common features and experiences of the condition that can encourage individuals to identify with others to benefit from the strength of an NF1 community. This strength could be utilized to enhance self-im-

age and general confidence. The basic assumptions of the disability rights movement, if internalized, could assist in focusing attention on the social, political,
economic, and environmental resources and recourses that have the potential to
assist individuals in varied dimensions of their lives.

IMPLICATIONS OF THE STUDY

A number of implications for family life and medical practice emerge from the
issues raised in the subjects' life narratives.

Family Support and Communication

*The one strongest message that emerges from subjects' life stories is the signifi-
cance of a strong supportive family in early life that imbued confidence and security
to the individual, usually before the NF1 was diagnosed or when that did occur, and
a family system that stood strongly by the individual and encouraged good coping
patterns to emerge.* Sharon, whose situation is described above, repeatedly referred
to parents who in her childhood actively and critically sought out the very best medical
care available, and to strongly supportive family members who were always "there
for her." In her recent periods of ill health her sisters and brothers-in-law accompanied
her on doctors' visits, entered into her decision-making about treatment options, and
were invariably at her bedside in the hospital during and following surgeries.

*For those who had a parent with NF1, the importance of positive parental
communication cannot be overemphasized.* Most affected adults with affected parents
did not have capable or inspiring role models in their parents. Their parents would not
talk to them about the potential practical or emotional issues around their NF1. Some
factors that may have explained their silence could have been the lack of knowledge
about NF1 and other genetic conditions twenty or more years ago, which may have
contributed to parents' feelings of fear and guilt, and sometimes to beliefs about
religious attribution. Secondly, parents frequently had suffered from significant
learning disorders, which engendered passive and tentative attitudes toward positive
communication or action. Thirdly, the climate for disclosure was very different from
today. The tendency of years past toward secrecy and shying away from open
communication about sensitive issues contrasts markedly with the emphasis in today's
society on open communication between family members and between intimates.
Most parents I interviewed who have affected children are making every effort to
educate them about their condition and to be available for their fears and concerns,
expressed or unexpressed. This may bode well for more informed and effective styles
of coping with NF1 in future generations.

Gender Considerations

NF1 may constitute an assault on the self-image and lifestyle of both men and
women because of its practical effects on (1) appearance, (2) educational career,

(3) earning ability and economic status, and (4) ability to reproduce without perceived danger. Although the most obvious complication of NF1, its effect on appearance, may hit women the hardest because of the cosmetic prescriptions of this society, this factor appears to be less significant than the other factors in the case of many subjects. In fact, neither the presence nor the absence of current tumors and other visible symptoms is a predictor of a satisfying or fulfilling life. In most cases of the older subjects, visible symptoms were not apparent until past the then-typical age for marriage. Visible symptoms of adult subjects could not in themselves explain childhood social exclusion except in very few cases.

Learning disabilities and related problems appear to be the chief mediating factor between subjects' NF1 and their past and current lifestyles and achievements. Learning disabilities may be more damaging to the developing male self-image than to that of the female, and in the company of other NF1 symptoms, impinge in more critical ways on male adult vocational and social aspirations and opportunities. While the number of cases described here is small it is significant that not one woman of the thirty-two in the sample withdrew from life's challenges in the manner that five of the twenty-two men did.

The implication that these men's surrender to NF1 came very early in their lives suggests that it may be even more imperative for parents to bolster the self-esteem and confidence level of affected male children and adolescents than those of affected female children, who some subjects speculate, may survive socially as adults through their ability to fantasize about their normalcy and their potential for social success and to strive heroically to meet these expectations.

Medical Practice

Some practitioners have described NF1 patients as "compliant," "gentle," "longing for acceptance," and "not embittered by their affliction" (for example, Trevisani et al. 1982). My interviews suggest that many affected persons do not fit these stereotypes. In fact, their statements to me reflect that they commonly are less than satisfied with their medical treatment and feel they have little access to health care providers who are genuinely interested in their patients' anxieties and concerns about their own or their children's conditions. If patients seem gentle or docile, I believe that this has been caused by the effects of learning disorders or other NF1-related, stress-creating factors that adversely impact personality, self-image, and coping abilities. Likewise, previous negative medical experiences have resulted cumulatively in their low expectations for medical care. For example, said Rachel, a highly educated and articulate woman who did not experience learning disorders, "It is hard to be aggressive and proactive. It takes effort; it takes time; it takes energy. And having had so many negative experiences, I feel like I've been conditioned into silence." Personality descriptions often appear to have been made anecdotally by clinicians who see patients briefly in physician-patient encounters, when patients may be extraordinarily anxious. Such encounters are not typical or neutral contexts for evaluating personality.

A number of suggestions for addressing patients' anxieties and needs emerges from their recounting of experiences and critical statements:

Addressing Anxiety

The great variability and unpredictability of NF1 symptoms have created a condition *without parameters*. The void resulting from the uncertainty around NF1 often creates a context of potential ever-present high anxiety in affected persons and their families that can involve every aspect of life, and particularly the medical. Within this context, any statements that doctors make may become sanctified and remembered long after the doctors' intentions. This is unfortunate because many statements appear to have been matter of fact, and often intended as tentative. Nonetheless, these statements, and particularly extreme ones given with the initial diagnosis, often have stayed with persons for many years after. Thus doctors often prematurely create their own parameters of *horror*. For example Terry had recounted the following incident:

He gave me a couple of prognoses like, "You'll be deaf by the time you're thirty and blind by the time you're forty." Very, very definite stuff like that. I was in a state of shock. I've never forgotten it.

While any of us might question a possible or even probable discrepancy between what was *said* and what was *intended* and what was *heard* and what was reported to *me* years after the fact, it is clear that *whatever* was said, the communications that did occur were often not ideal. Patients left in a state of anxiety and with very little understanding of their conditions.

There is an old dictum, "Never be the bearer of bad news." If the recipient does not like the message he or she may literally shoot the messenger. This may also be done symbolically, by remembering the nature and content of the informing interaction bitterly or at least negatively. Since doctors are often the bearers of bad news, particular thought should be given as to how to accomplish the task effectively, yet gently. Particularly for breaking such news as the initial diagnosis of NF1, and more so because of the great uncertainty that is involved, it is imperative to cushion the giving of diagnoses or prognoses with great care and sensitivity.

The doctor can provide a realistic context of expectation for the most frightening prognoses, for example the chances of a child or adult developing a brain tumor or becoming blind or deaf. *Because of the unpredictability of NF1, patients may be more sensitive to a doctor's every literal word than are patients with more benign or predictable conditions. Therefore doctors should be aware of the potency of their statements and the particular need for clear and supportive communications. The greatest gift the doctor can give is time—time for explanation, for the patient's ventilation, and for answering questions.* This suggestion is made with full knowledge of the ever-increasing strictures on time being imposed by "managed care."

Nonetheless, if clinical care is to be optimum, or even reasonable, there is little way to cut short the time needed for adequate communication.

Because patients may be so shocked at the initial disclosure, they may not adequately be able to formulate the many questions that may plague them during the following hours or days. The routine scheduling of a follow-up appointment would allow them the opportunity to ask for more information, and at this second visit answers to their questions may be more absorbable and hence useful for their understanding and planning. Also, if need be, the doctor may be able to get more information in the interim to share with the patient. Further, the patient may wish to arrange for a spouse, family member, or other support companions to accompany them on this next visit. This second appointment should follow soon after the initial disclosure. The doctor might also routinely refer the patient to a geneticist and/or genetic counselor to explain some of the many issues around their complex condition and also discuss reproductive issues if appropriate. Those few persons in this study who were sent to or did find their way to geneticists or genetic counselors found these specialists to be extremely helpful.

Doctors could give cognizance to the realities of patients' anxieties by asking them how they feel about specific issues or even about their NF1 in general. One subject commented that in a long history of medical problems and treatment, only one doctor had ever asked her how she felt about having NF1. Although this was a resident in training who visited her bedside but never actually contributed to her clinical treatment, she remembered this incident from seventeen years before as a rare human expression of caring by a doctor. Indeed, in the case of a condition like NF1, where there is no cure and often no treatment for specific symptoms, the traditional "bedside manner" may be more substantively important than focused clinical care.

Needs of Adults—Total Life Cycle Focus

While pediatricians are best placed to serve as case managers for the treatment of children, and this hopefully happens, in the case of adults many fall through the cracks. These adults sorely need a centrally coordinated medical service with doctors sophisticated with or at least familiar with NF1 to assess and treat their problems. *Adults with NF1, as well as adults with other genetic disorders, often feel they are the forgotten ones while medical interest and attention tends to go to children.* Many of the genetics clinics organized for NF1 and other conditions see only children except when they see young adults for genetic counseling. These clinics do not have the specialists readily available to assess adults. Likewise speaker topics and discussions at support group meetings most frequently center on the problems of children.

One subject entering middle age reported that her internist and neurologist, while doctors she respects and likes, do not know what special issues she might encounter as an adult with NF1. They told her they will watch her carefully, but do not themselves know what to expect. Adults have reported to me a variety of questions they asked their doctors such as, "What are the implications of hormone replacement therapy for a woman with NF1?" because they recognize the significance of changing hormonal levels at earlier life periods. Or, "Will menopause bring other issues to be addressed?" These are a few of many questions that persons with NF1 are asking as they age, and they get few answers from their regular doctors.

Comprehensive NF1 services should give attention to the learning and social deficits of adults. Just as NF clinics regularly have psychologists, speech therapists, and other specialists available to test children and advise parents about their child's learning disabilities and related problems, there should also be such specialists available for adults. Social deficits that developed many years ago have often continued into adulthood and should be addressed. Interventions might assist in the mastering of social skills, providing assertiveness training, or general image-enhancing therapy. Workshops or support groups to assist in preparation for employment would ideally be a component of such services. Subjects have also suggested that cosmetic make-up specialists and even fashion consultants knowledgeable about the cosmetic issues of NF1 be available for consultation. Such assistance could address the nagging concerns about appearance that beleaguer many persons, contributing to problems of poor self-image.

Continuity of Care

A serious problem that I have observed for both affected adults and children is the *frequent absence of continuity of care.* In the case of a condition that may require the services of many specialists for adequate treatment, patients sometimes seem to see doctors almost helter-skelter, by luck, or when harried mothers or adults remember to go in, or can get appointments. This appears to be true of both those who see private practitioners and those who belong to HMOs.

The situation is exacerbated by inordinately long waiting periods for appointments, patients' lack of sophistication about the procedures for service, and passivity often born of feelings of hopelessness or having had previous negative medical experiences. My interviews suggest that patients at the largest HMOs may receive the most unsatisfactory care unless they are educated and aggressive, even though the potential is there for reasonable continuity of care. Where the situation should be "refer and remember," it is usually "refer and forget."

Support Groups

Subjects' accounts underline the helpfulness of NF and other support groups for many persons. Those who attend support groups and medical conferences sponsored by the national and local NF organizations are made aware of the "state of the science" advances and have better access to clinicians familiar with the condition. They can learn from the experiences of others. The potential for self-image and attitude enhancement that NF support groups may offer was discussed above. It is important for doctors to become acquainted with relevant support groups in their area to which they might refer patients. In most metropolitan areas there are support groups for children and adults with learning disorders, as well as for many other special health conditions related to NF1. Specialized resources are listed in Appendix IV.

Through the sharing of their experiences, hopes, dreams, and fears with me, the persons whose life stories form the basis of this volume have deepened and broadened my understandings of human needs and desires and joys and sorrows, and made vividly alive the meanings of the condition with which they must live alone. Rachel's thoughtful statement embodies the complexities of the sadness and hopefulness of living with NF1:

The NF is a powerful tool that keeps me conscious. It's helped me to realize that the tumors stop at one point, and the scarring stops at one point, and the cafe-au-lait map stops at one point. And I can actually break through them. It's not easy; it's a struggle, and it's a challenge. But I can actually weave my way through them and to the Me. You know, the person inside, that soul center which everyone has. People who are dwarfs have it; people who are in wheelchairs have it; even normal folk walking around the world have it. You can actually give it out to somebody who will then take it, and caress it, and love it.

Appendix I:
Neurofibromatosis 1

The diagnosis of NF1 is based on clinical criteria. In 1987 the Consensus Development Conference on Neurofibromatosis was convened by the National Institute of Neurological and Communicative Disorders and Stroke, the National Cancer Institute, and the National Institutes of Health Office of Medical Applications of Research to address varied issues concerning the diagnosis and treatment of the neurofibromatoses. The consensus panel proposed that a diagnosis of NF1 be based on an individual exhibiting two or more of the following features:

Six or more cafe-au-lait macules over 5 millimeters in greatest diameter in prepubertal individuals and over 15 millimeters in greatest diameter in postpubertal individuals

Two or more neurofibromas of any type or one plexiform neurofibroma

Freckling in the axillary or inguinal regions [armpit and/or groin]

Optic glioma

Two or more Lisch Nodules (iris hamartomas)

A distinctive osseous lesion such as sphenoid dysplasia or thinning of long bone cortex with or without pseudoarthrosis

A first-degree relative (parent, sibling, or offspring) with NF1 by the above criteria (National Institutes of Health 1988. Also update, Gutmann et al. 1997)

The physical features of NF1 may develop and be apparent in different periods of life. For instance, cafe-au-lait spots become apparent in early childhood. Lisch Nodules (clumps of pigment on the iris) develop in late childhood. These do not in themselves cause problems. They are present in 95 percent of persons with NF, and for this reason ophthalmologic examinations are typically carried out on persons suspected of having NF1. Lisch Nodules are visible only when viewed through a slit lamp. Neurofibromas, the most common feature associated with NF1, tend to appear after adolescence and often increase in number through the life span. Most neurofibromas are small soft nodules on or just under the skin. Those inside the body are more potentially problematic than cutaneous ones and may pose a threat to health, mobility, and even life.

Some of the most serious complications of NF1 are manifest early in childhood. Optic gliomas, tumors causing thickening of the optic nerve and complications of the eye socket and lid, tend to be apparent in early childhood. These tumors are suggested to occur in about 15 percent of children with NF1, as detected by Magnetic Resonance Imaging scans (MRIs), but in most cases these tumors will not affect the vision or be apparent (Listernick et al. 1989). Skeletal abnormalities such as scoliosis, kyphosis, or pseudoarthrosis—the thinning, bowing, and sometimes breaking of the tibia—likewise tend to be apparent in early childhood and should be monitored and treated aggressively with bracing or surgery. It is estimated that some 10 percent of persons with NF1 have structural scoliosis (Akbarnia et al. 1992). Plexiform neurofibromas, large tumors that occur in about one-quarter of cases, in rare instances constitute the most potentially unsightly feature of NF1. When they occur they are apparent in infancy or early childhood and may require aggressive and complex surgeries. These more noticeable plexiform neurofibromas tend to be apparent by age five or younger and if they do not appear by late childhood will not be a problem later in life. Riccardi (1992:214) suggests that there is a lifetime risk for NF1-related malignancy of about 5 percent over the general population risk, which he states to be about 25 percent.

Following diagnosis (which may occur at any point in life), appropriate follow-up is essential. For most persons this may constitute regular thorough interviewing and examination by a general pediatrician or internist. For persons with suspected complications, appropriate care may necessitate the attentions of a neurologist, dermatologist, orthopedist, ophthalmologist, geneticist, plastic surgeon, speech and/or hearing specialist, and/or social service personnel to assist with psychosocial and/or economic concerns. NF clinics have been opened at many major urban medical centers and these have available many specialists familiar with the problems of NF1. (See Appendix IV.)

Korf (1990:25) has noted:

NF is a disorder, not a disease and most people who are affected are healthy. Yet in spite of this, many affected individuals cannot escape a greater-than-average awareness of the fragility of life. Living with NF calls for inner strength, support from family and friends, as well as alert medical care.

COGNITIVE ASPECTS OF NF1 AND LEARNING DISORDERS

A significant literature has developed on varied cognitive aspects of NF1, particularly centering on learning disabilities and related problems of children. For a comprehensive statement see North et al. 1997. Studies have reported that up to 50 percent of children with NF1 exhibit some form of learning disability (Mouridsen and Sorensen 1995). This figure constitutes five times the frequency that is found in the general population (Aron et al. 1990). A child is considered to have a learning disability when he/she exhibits normal intellectual potential but still has great difficulty in accomplishing the normal learning tasks of school.

Learning and Related Disabilities

During the past decade researchers have attempted to define the profile of NF1-related learning disabilities. Studies with small, but well controlled samples of children with NF1 and their siblings have reported that in studies comparing affected children with nonaffected siblings, subjects with NF1 have tested with lower ranges of IQ and have exhibited significant learning disabilities in written language and reading and in neuromotor dysfunction as compared with their siblings (Hofman et al. 1994). Dilts et al. (1996) reported that children with NF1 were found to be less competent than their siblings on measures of cognitive, language, and motor development, visual-spacial judgment, visual-motor integration, and academic achievement. Preliminary evaluations revealed that more children with NF1 than matched controls were in need of special education. The authors note that children with NF1 with special needs, particularly in the areas of oral and written language, may be underidentified in the schools. (See also Denckla 1996.)

Aron et al. (1990) concluded that three forms of learning disabilities are common in children with NF1:

1. A specific learning problem that is confined to reading, writing, calculating, or a combination of these skills.
2. Lack of coordination in varying degrees, most frequently in fine motor coordination in activities like holding a pencil or pen, tying shoelaces, or buttoning or unbuttoning.
3. Hyperactivity, distractibility, and variable attention span, today commonly called "attention deficit disorder."

Eliason (1988) reported from a study sample of children with NF1 compared to a matched sample of learning-disordered students without NF1 that NF1 children are less likely to present verbal language or memory problems that primarily affect reading. Further, children with NF1 are more likely to display nonverbal learning problems that affect written language and organization skills. Eliason (1988) notes:

Nonverbal types of learning disability are less likely to be recognized as forms of LD [learning disability] because they have a lesser effect on academic achievement and they have behavioral components that may be more striking than the cognitive deficits. Two behavioral features of visual-perceptual disability are impulsivity and social imperception.

Elsewhere, Eliason (1986), from another study sample that included some of the children in the above study, commented further on impulsivity and social imperception:

Impulsivity refers to a behavioral style of acting quickly without considering the consequences of an act. Social imperception refers to an inability to perceive and interpret social cues in the environment, such as facial expressions, tone of voice, posture, and gestures. The child with social imperception may violate personal space by standing or sitting too close to others, and has difficulty perceiving when others are angry or displeased with them. The combination of impulsivity and social imperception is often misinterpreted as "hyperactivity." Indeed, nearly one-half of these NF children had been diagnosed as "hyperactive" or as having an attention deficit disorder, and eight of the twenty-three were taking stimulant medications. Mothers described these children as highly unpredictable, impulsive, and socially inept.

For valuable discussions of the above subjects see various papers in the collection *Childhood Learning Disabilities in Neurofibromatosis* (National Neurofibromatosis Foundation, Inc. 1988). Denckla's article in this collection (1988) presents readable expositions of core problems and also suggestions for assisting children at home with their schoolwork and social, interactional, and organizational problems.

The current problems reported by adults in my study are consistent with the findings of Lewandowski and Arcangelo (1994) who report from a review of the literature on social adjustment and self concept of adults with learning disabilities that the strongest findings are feelings of insecurity and inadequacy and lowered measured self-concept, presumably due to years of educational failure and social difficulties.

Denckla (1993) has pointed up some of the problems of adults with the nonverbal learning disabilities commonly attributed to many children with NF1. These persons exhibit "executive dysfunction," pertaining to the executor system within the brain that engages in more advanced and future-oriented processes. Further they often are characterized as "*spacy*" or "*disorganized in a disoriented way* [Denckla's italics]." They may have problems seeing the "big picture," rather than details. "Despite good verbal skills, they write poorly because they do not summarize, overview, or relate pieces of information." They may not get the "main idea" (p. 118). Denckla suggests these persons may need social cognitive training in social skills to make them more perceptive of the "messages conveyed by the faces, postures, and vocal tones of others" (p. 120).

HISTORY OF NF1

Various researchers suggest that NF1 was identified in writing and in graphic portrayals in second-, thirteenth-, fifteenth-, and sixteenth-century drawings. Zanca and Zanca (1980) claim that the earliest clinical case description was by an Italian physician and naturalist in the sixteenth century. Quasimodo of the *Hunchback of*

Notre Dame by Victor Hugo, first published in 1831, is thought to have had NF1 (Solomon 1968). A number of eighteenth- and nineteenth-century medical descriptions exist, and an 1849 review of the literature cited seventy-five references. The first clearly definitive work, *Ueber die Multiplen Fibrome der Haut und ihre Beziehung zu den multiplen Neuromen* [*On Multiple Neurofibromas of the Skin and Their Relationship to Multiple Neuromas*], was published by Friederich Daniel von Recklinghausen in 1882. In this volume, which is based on two cases, von Recklinghausen cited 168 citations of prior publications and described cutaneous tumors as deriving from peripheral nerves. Thenceforth the condition became widely known as von Recklinghausen's Disease. The end of the nineteenth century saw a burgeoning of literature on NF1 and the condition won wide medical attention. For more detailed historical discussions, see Mulvihill (1990) and Huson (1994b).

NF became known to the contemporary general public through its association with The Elephant Man's Disease, the severe health condition of Joseph Merrick. As detailed in Chapter 11, Sir Frederick Treves brought Merrick to London Hospital in 1884 and there publicized his case. He labeled Merrick "A Case of Congenital Deformity" in an 1885 article. Eminent dermatologists Crocker in 1905 and Weber in 1909 first suggested that Merrick had neurofibromatosis. In 1982 the suggestion was challenged by several clinicians who proposed that he had three diseases. In 1986 two Canadian geneticists called the condition "Proteus syndrome," a newly recognized and considerably more severe condition than NF1 (Tibbles and Cohen 1986; Cohen 1988). This diagnosis is still under discussion. However, it is now generally conceded that The Elephant Man's Disease was not neurofibromatosis. For arguments on this issue see Seward (1994) and Clark (1994).

Appendix II:
The Sample

AGE

Years Old	Number of Subjects
19–29	3
30–39	23
40–49	13
50–59	9
60 +	6
Total	54

EDUCATION

Less than high school graduation	1
High school graduation	18
Courses taken in four-year colleges, two-year community colleges, or specialized business or art schools	23
Community college graduation	1
Four-year B.A. or B.S. graduation	6
M.A. completion	3
Ph.D. course work	2
Total	54

MARITAL STATUS

Marital status varied between men and women. Women have married much more frequently than men. Of the thirty-two women that I interviewed, twenty, about two-thirds, were currently married and five were divorced. Seven, or less than one-fourth, never married. This profile is quite different from that of the males. Of twenty-two males, ten, less than one-half, were married; two were divorced; and another ten had never married. While these numbers are small, the subjects were all recruited in the same manner, and the visibility and severity of their NF1 conditions are comparable.

	Women	Men
Married	20	10
Single	12	12
(Divorced	5	2)
Total	32	22

VISIBILITY

I rated individuals as to their visibility and severity. My visibility ratings of mild, moderate, or severe, were based on the appearance of the person fully dressed and how readily symptoms could be perceived in impersonal interactions. It should be noted, however, that many persons who display no tumors on areas visible when wearing normal street clothes have numerous tumors or cafe-au-lait (darkened) spots on the torso that would be apparent in physically intimate situations, and may gravely affect sexual behavior.

1. *Mild*   Few visible tumors outside of normal clothing areas; gait and posture appear unremarkable when casually observed (this allows for heavy coating of neurofibromas on the body and some minor skeletal symptoms).

2. *Moderate* Some tumors on neck, face, hands, mild scoliosis or other skeletal feature without noticeable limp.

3. *Severe*   Numerous tumors on face, optic glioma (tumor) that has affected sight and eye socket, severe scoliosis or skeletal features with noticeable limp.

Visibility

Mild	17
Moderate	19
Severe	18
Total	54

SEVERITY

My severity ratings of mild, moderate, or severe were based on a combination of clinical and cosmetic implications that may potentially affect lifestyle, mobility, and/or threaten life.

1. *Mild*   Symptoms such as neurofibromas or mild learning disorders that do not threaten physical or social life.

2. *Moderate*   Symptoms may compromise lifestyle but are not severely threatening. Numerous external or internal neurofibromas, mild scoliosis, controlled learning disorders.

3. *Severe*   Hundreds or thousands of visible neurofibromas that threaten functioning; blinding optic glioma; severe scoliosis or other skeletal features; serious internal neurofibromas; or malignancies. Serious emotional or psychological problems associated with learning disorders or lifestyle issues.

Severity

Severity	
Mild	30
Moderate	10
Severe	<u>14</u>
Total	<u>54</u>

Six persons died during the period of interviewing (three women and three men). Two women died from breast cancer, and the third woman from an embolism. Two men died from NF-related brain tumors, and the third man from a heart attack, apparently related to his many surgeries and heavy medications for controlling his tumor-driven pain.

Appendix III:
The Voices

The lived experience of NF1 has been told through the voices of many subjects who shared with me incidents and thoughts that they typically had never talked about with another person before. Below are listed the persons most frequently quoted. Included here are their ages at the beginning of the interview period, occupations, learning disabilities (LD) if present, their educational attainment, degree of visibility and severity of NF1, and if married and if with children. These features are presented in general terms to protect the confidentiality of participants.

Benjamin   Thirty-five-year-old on disability. Formerly retail manager. LD. College graduate. Mildly visible and severely affected. Benjamin died during interview period.

Carrie   African-American thirty-seven-year-old on disability for many years. Severe LD. High school dropout. Mildly visible and severely affected. Unmarried with one child and one grandchild.

Cecilia   Thirty-two-year-old gymnastics instructor. College graduate. Moderately visible and mildly affected.

Chuck   Thirty-five-year-old salesman. LD. Some college courses. Nonvisible and severely affected.

Elise   Forty-two-year-old clerical worker. LD. Some college courses. Mildly visible and moderately affected. Married with children.

Florence   Sixty-year-old high school teacher. College graduate. Moderately visible and mildly affected. Married with children and grandchildren.

Grace   Fifty-three-year-old service worker. LD. Highly visible and moderately affected. Divorced with children.

Hal	Thirty-year-old part-time clerical worker. LD. Some college courses. Moderately visible and severely affected.
Harry	Forty-two-year-old counselor for disabled student services. LD. College graduate. Highly visible and severely affected.
Isabelle	Fifty-eight-year-old on disability. Former service worker. Married with children. Quadriplegic. Very seriously affected.
Jim	Forty-five-year-old security guard. LD. Some college courses. Moderately visible and severely affected.
Jody	Thirty-eight-year-old high school teacher. College graduate. Mildly visible and mildly affected. Married with children.
Lou	Forty-year-old on disability. Formally clerical worker. LD. High school graduate. Highly visible and severely affected. Divorced with children. Lou died during interview period.
Michael	Thirty-five-year-old service worker. LD. Some college courses. Moderately visible and mildly affected. Married with children.
Nathan	Thirty-five-year-old clerical worker. LD. College graduate. Very visible and severely affected. Nathan died during interview period.
Norita	Latina twenty-eight-year-old teacher's aide. LD. Some college courses. Moderately visible and moderately affected.
Peter	Thirty-year-old factory worker. LD. Some college courses. Mildly visible and mildly affected. Married with children.
Rachel	Thirty-five-year-old educational researcher. College and graduate degrees. Moderately visible and moderately affected.
Randy	Twenty-six-year-old clerical worker. LD. Some college courses. Nonvisible and severely affected.
Reggie	Forty-three-year-old professional. College graduate. Mildly visible and mildly affected. Married.
Rhoda	Sixty-two-year-old retired clerical worker. LD. Business school. Nonvisible and mildly affected. Married with children.
Robbie	Thirty-four-year-old clerical worker. LD. College graduate. Highly visible and severely affected.
Rosa	Nineteen-year-old college student and clerical worker. Highly visible and moderately affected. Married during interview period.
Rudy	Forty-year-old service worker. College graduate. Highly visible and moderately affected.
Sarah	Thirty-eight-year-old clerical worker. LD. Some college courses. Moderately visible and severely affected. Married with child.
Sharon	Forty-five-year-old financial analyst. LD. Some college courses. Very visible and severely affected.
Terry	Thirty-two-year-old on disability. Formally office manager. LD. College and graduate degrees. Nonvisible but severely affected.

Theresa   Latina fifty-seven-year-old office manager. High school graduate. Moder-
            ately visible and mildly affected. Married with children and grandchildren.
Victor   Thirty-year-old factory worker. LD. Some college courses. Mildly visible
            and mildly affected. Married with children.

Appendix IV:
Resources

1. National Neurofibromatosis Foundation, Inc. (NNFF)
Thirty-two chapters throughout the country. Call for information about NF clinics nationally.

95 Pine Street, 16th Floor
New York, NY 10005
Tel: (800) 323–7938 or (212) 344–NNFF
Fax: (212) 747–0004
E-mail: NNFF@aol.com
Website: www.nf.org

2. Neurofibromatosis, Inc. (NF, Inc.)
Nine chapters. Call for information about independent local support groups in various states.

8855 Annapolis Road, Suite 110
Lanham, MD 20706–2924
Tel: (800) 942–6825 or (301) 577–8984
Fax: (301) 577–0016
E-mail: NFInc1@aol.com
Website: www.nfinc.org

3. The Alliance of Genetic Support Groups
Call for information about numerous support groups, services, and resources.

4301 Connecticut Avenue NW, Suite 404
Washington, DC 20008–2304

Tel: (800) 336–GENE or (202) 966–5557
Fax: (202) 966–8553
E-mail: info@geneticalliance.org
Website: www.geneticalliance.org

4. **National Society of Genetic Counselors**
   Call for referrals and general information.

   233 Canterbury Drive
   Wallingford, PA 19086–6617
   Tel: (610) 872–7608
   Fax: (610) 872–1192
   E-mail: NSGC@aol.com
   Website: www.NSGC.org

5. **The Neurofibromatosis Association (United Kingdom)**
   Call for information about resources in the United Kingdom and Europe

   82 London Road
   Kingston on Thames
   Surrey KT2 6PX
   Tel: 0181 547 1636
   Fax: 0181 974 5601
   E-mail: nfa@zetnet.co.uk
   Website: www.nfa.zetnet.co.uk

References

Ablon, Joan
   1984   Little People in America: The Social Dimensions of Dwarfism. New York: Praeger Publishers.
   1988   Living with Difference: Families with Dwarf Children. New York: Praeger Publishers.
   1992a   Intangibles: The Psychologic Implications of Uncertainty, Diagnosis, Chronicity, and Prognosis in NF. *In* Psychosocial Aspects of the Neurofibromatoses: Impact on the Individual, Impact on the Family. Pp. 49–64. Jane Novak Pugh Conference Series. Vol. 3. New York: The National Neurofibromatosis Foundation, Inc.
   1992b   The Social Dimensions of Genetic Disorder. Practicing Anthropology 14(1): 10–13.
   1995   "The Elephant Man" as "Self" and "Other": The Psycho-social Costs of a Misdiagnosis. Social Science and Medicine 40(11):1481–1489.
   1996   Gender Response to Neurofibromatosis 1. Social Science and Medicine 42(1):99–109.
   1998   Coping with Visible and Invisible Stigma: Neurofibromatosis 1. *In* Accessing the Issues: Current Research in Disability Studies. Elaine Makas, Beth Haller, and Tanis Doe, eds. Pp. 45–49. Lewiston, ME: The Society for Disability Studies. Edmund S. Muskie Institute of Public Affairs.
Adams, P. F., and V. Benson
   1991   Current Estimates from the National Health Interview Survey, 1990. Vital Health Statistics 10(181):1–212.
Akbarnia, B. A., K. R. Gabriel and E. Beckman
   1992   Prevalence of Scoliosis in Neurofibromatosis. Spine 17(8S):S244–S248.
American Medical News
   1981   20 February.

Aron, Alan M., Allan E. Rubenstein, Sibylle A. Wallace, and Jane C. Halperin
  1990   Learning Disabilities in Neurofibromatosis. *In* Neurofibromatosis: A Hand-
                    book for Patients, Families and Health-Care Professionals. A. Rubenstein
                    and B. Korf, eds. Pp. 55–58. New York: Thieme Medical Publishers.
Asch, Adrienne
  1996   Genetics and Employment; More Disability Discrimination. *In* The Human
                    Genome Project and the Future of Health Care. Thomas H. Murray, Mark
                    A. Rothstein, and Robert F. Murry, Jr., eds. Pp. 158–172. Bloomington and
                    Indianapolis, IN: Indiana University Press.
Asch, Adrienne, and Michelle Fine
  1988   Shared Dreams: A Left Perspective on Disability Rights and Reproductive
                    Rights. *In* Women with Disabilities: Essays in Psychology, Culture, and
                    Politics. Michelle Fine and Adrienne Asch, eds. Pp. 297–305. Philadelphia,
                    PA: Temple University Press.
Asch, Adrienne, and Gail Geller
  1996   Feminism, Bioethics, and Genetics. *In* Feminism and Bioethics: Beyond
                    Reproduction. Susan M. Wolf, ed. Pp. 318–350. New York: Oxford Uni-
                    versity Press.
Benjamin, C. M., A. Colley, D. Donnai, H. Kingston, R. Harris, and L. Kerzin-Storrar
  1993   Neurofibromatosis Type 1 (NF1): Knowledge, Experience, and Reproduc-
                    tive Decisions of Affected Patients and Families. Journal of Medical Ge-
                    netics 30:567–574.
Bobinski, Mary Anne
  1996   Genetics and Reproductive Decision Making. *In* The Human Genome
                    Project and the Future of Health Care. Thomas H. Murray, Mark A.
                    Rothstein, and Robert F. Murry, Jr., eds. Pp. 79–112. Bloomington and
                    Indianapolis, IN: Indiana University Press.
Boutté, Marie
  1987   The Stumbling Disease: A Case Study of Stigma among Asorean-Portu-
                    guese. Social Science and Medicine 24:209–217.
  1990   Waiting for the Family Legacy: The Experience of Being At Risk for
                    Machado-Josephs Disease. Social Science and Medicine 30(8):839–847.
Breslau, N.
  1985   Psychiatric Disorder in Children with Physical Disabilities. American
                    Academy of Child Psychiatry 24:148–149.
Brown, Dale S.
  1994   Working Effectively with People Who Have Learning Disabilities and
                    Attention Deficit Hyperactivity Disorder. Program on Employment and
                    Disability. New York: Cornell University Press.
Carey, John C.
  1988   Neurofibromatosis Is Not The Elephant Man's Disease. National Neurofi-
                    bromatosis Foundation. Newsletter 10:3.
  1990a   The Genetics of Neurofibromatosis. *In* Neurofibromatosis: A Handbook
                    for Patients, Families, and Health Care Professionals. A. Rubenstein and B.
                    Korf, eds. Pp. 163–224. New York: Thieme Medical Publishers Inc.
  1990b   Personal Communication, 16 May.

Clark, R. D.
  1994   Proteus Syndrome. *In* The Neurofibromatoses: A Pathogenic and Clinical
                  Overviews. S. M. Huson and R. A. C. Hughes, eds. Pp. 402–414. London:
                  Chapman and Hall Medical.
Cohen, M., Jr.
  1988   Understanding Proteus Syndrome, Unmasking the Elephant Man, and
                  Stemming Elephant Fever. Neurofibromatosis 1:260.
Collins, Francis
  1991   Personal Communication, 14 January.
  1998   Contemplating the Completion of the Human Genome Sequence, Public
                  Lecture, University of California, San Francisco, 19 October.
Collins, Francis S., and Leslie Fink
  1995   The Human Genome Project. Alcohol, Health and Research World
                  19(3):190–195.
Counterman, April Porter, Saylor F. Conway, and Shashidhar Pai
  1995   Psychological Adjustment of Children and Adolescents With Neurofibro-
                  matosis. Children's Health Care (24)4:223–234.
Cranor, Carl F., ed.
  1994   Are Genes Us? The Social Consequences of the New Genetics. New
                  Brunswick, NJ: Rutgers University Press.
Csapo, M.
  1991   Psychosocial Adjustment of Children with Short Stature: Social Compe-
                  tence, Behavior Problems, Self-esteem, Family Functioning, Body Image,
                  and Reaction to Frustrations. Behavioral Disorders 16:219–224.
Davis, Lennard J., ed.
  1997   The Disability Studies Reader. New York: Routledge.
Denckla, Martha B.
  1988   Helping Children with Non-Verbal Learning Disabilities Outside of School.
                  In Childhood Learning Disabilities in Neurofibromatosis, Pp. 3–25. Con-
                  ference Series Volume 1. New York: The National Neurofibromatosis
                  Foundation, Inc.
  1993   The Child with Developmental Disabilities Grown Up: Adult Residua of
                  Childhood Disorders. Behavioral Neurology 11(1):105.
  1996   Neurofibromatosis Type 1: A Model for the Pathogenesis of Reading
                  Disability. Mental Retardation and Developmental Disabilities Research
                  Reviews: 2:48–53. New York: Wiley-Liss.
Dilts, Constance, John C. Carey, John C. Kircher, Robert O. Hoffman, Donnell Creel,
Kenneth Ward, Elaine Clark, and Claire O. Leonard
  1996   Children and Adolescents with Neurofibromatosis 1: A Behavioral Pheno-
                  type. Developmental and Behavioral Pediatrics 17(4):229–239.
Drimmer, F.
  1985   The Elephant Man. New York: G. P. Putnam's Sons.
Eisenberg, M.
  1982   Disability as Stigma. *In* Disabled People as Second-Class Citizens. M.
                  Eisenberg, C. Griggins, and R. Duval, eds. Pp 3–12. New York: Springer
                  Publishing Company.

Eisenberg, M., C. Griggins, and R. Duval, eds.
    1982   Disabled People as Second-Class Citizens. New York: Springer Publishing
                    Company.
Eliason, Michelle J.
    1986   Neurofibromatosis: Implications for Learning and Behavior. Developmen-
                    tal and Behavioral Pediatrics 7(3):175–179.
    1988   Neuropsychological Patterns: Neurofibromatosis Compared to Develop-
                    mental Learning Disorders. Neurofibromatosis 1:17–25.
Ellis, Sarah A.
    1990   Psychosocial Aspects of Appearance in Neurofibromatosis. *In* Neurofibro-
                    matosis: A Handbook for Patients, Families, and Health Care Professionals.
                    A. Rubenstein and B. Korf, eds. Pp. 225–230. New York: Thieme Medical
                    Publishers Inc.
Ferner, R. E.
    1994   Intellect in Neurofibromatosis 1. *In* The Neurofibromatoses: A Pathogenic
                    and Clinical Overview, S. M. Huson and R.A.C. Hughes, eds. Pp. 233–254.
                    London: Chapman and Hall Medical.
Fine, Michelle, and Adrienne Asch
    1985   Disabled Women: Sexism without the Pedestal. *In* Women and Disability:
                    The Double Handicap. M. J. Deegan and N. A. Brooks, eds. Pp. 6–22. New
                    Brunswick, NJ: Transaction Books.
    1988   Women with Disabilities: Essays in Psychology, Culture and Politics.
                    Philadelphia: Temple University Press.
Finger, Anne
    1992   Claiming All of Our Bodies: Reproductive Rights and Disability. *In* Femi-
                    nist Philosophies: Problems, Theories, and Applications. Janet A. Kourany,
                    James P. Sterba, and Rosemarie Tong, eds. Pp. 87–94. Englewood Cliffs,
                    NJ: Prentice-Hall.
Fortier, Laurie M., and Richard L. Wanlass
    1984   Family Crises Following the Diagnosis of a Handicapped Child. Family
                    Relations 33:13–24.
Gelehrter, Thomas, and Francis S. Collins
    1990   Principles of Medical Genetics. Baltimore: Williams and Wilkins.
Gilligan, C.
    1982   In a Different Voice. Cambridge, MA: Harvard University Press.
Goffman, Irving
    1963   Stigma: Notes on the Management of Spoiled Identity. Englewood Cliffs,
                    NJ: Prentice-Hall.
Gostin, Larry
    1994   Genetic Discrimination: The Use of Genetically Based Diagnostic and
                    Prognostic Tests by Employers and Insurers. *In* Genes and Human Self-
                    Knowledge: Historical and Philosophical Reflections on Modern Genetics.
                    Robert F. Weir, Susan C. Lawrence, and Evan Fales, eds. Pp. 12–163. Iowa
                    City: University of Iowa Press.
Graham, J., and A. Kligman
    1985   The Psychology of Cosmetic Treatment. New York: Praeger Publishers.

Graham, Peter W., and Fritz H. Oehlschlaeger
1992   Articulating the Elephant Man: Joseph Merrick and His Interpreters. Baltimore: The Johns Hopkins University Press.

Grealy, Lucy
1994   Autobiography of a Face. Boston: Houghton Mifflin.

Gutmann, David H., Arthur Aylsworth, John C. Carey, Bruce Korf, Joan Marks, Reed E. Pyeritz, Allan Rubenstein, and David Viskochil
1997   The Diagnostic Evaluation and Multidisciplinary Management of Neurofibromatosis 1 and Neurofibromatosis 2. Journal of the American Medical Association 278 (1):51–57.

Hahn, Harlan
1988   The Politics of Physical Differences: Disability and Discrimination. Journal of Social Issues 44(1):39–47.

Hall, Judith G.
1988   The Value of the Study of Natural History in Genetic Disorders and Congenital Anomaly Syndrome. Journal of Medical Genetics 25:434–444.
1990a   Nontraditional Inheritance. Growth/Genetics and Hormones 6(4):1–4.
1990b   Genomic Imprinting: Review and Relevance to Human Diseases, American Journal of Human Genetics 46:857–873.

Hanna, William John, and Betsy Rogovsky
1993   Women with Disabilities: Two Handicaps Plus. *In* Perspectives on Disability, 2nd ed. M. Nagler, ed. Pp. 109–120. Palo Alto: Health Markets Research. [Originally published in Disability, Handicap and Society 6(1) 1991: 49–63].

Hatfield, E., and S. Sprecher
1986   Mirror, Mirror . . . The Importance of Looks in Everyday Life. Albany: State University of New York Press.

Heim, Ruth A., Lauren N.W. Kam-Morgan, Cameron G. Binnie, David D. Corns, Matthew C. Cayouette, Rosann A. Farber, Arthur S. Aylsworth, Lawrence M. Silverman, and Michael C. Luce
1995   Distribution of 13 Truncating Mutations in The Neurofibromatosis 1 Gene. Human Molecular Genetics (4)6:975–981.

Helander, Einar
1993   Prejudice and Dignity: An Introduction to Community-based Rehabilitation. United Nations Development Program Report No. E93-III-B.3. New York: United Nations Development Program.

Hofman, Karen J., Emily Harris, Nick Bryan, and Martha B. Denckla
1994   Neurofibromatosis Type 1: The Cognitive Phenotype. Journal of Pediatrics 124:81–88.

Howe, Louisa
1964   The Concept of Community: Some Impolications for the Development of Community Psychiatry. *In* Handbook of Community Psychiatry and Community Mental Health. L. Bellak, ed. Pp. 16–46. New York and London: Grune & Stratton.

Howell, M., and P. Ford
1980   The True History of the Elephant Man. New York: Penguin Books.

Huson, S. M.
   1994a   Neurofibromatosis 1: A Clinical and Genetic Overview. *In* The Neurofibro-
                  matoses: A Pathogenic and Clinical Overview. S. M. Huson and R.A.C.
                  Hughes, eds. Pp. 160–203. London: Chapman and Hall Medical.
   1994b   Neurofibromatosis: Historical Perspective, Classification and Diagnostic
                  Criteria. *In* The Neurofibromatoses: A Pathogenic and Clinical Overview.
                  S. M. Huson and R.A.C. Hughes, eds. Pp. 1–23. London: Chapman and
                  Hall Medical.
Huson, S. M., and R.A.C. Hughes, eds.
   1994   The Neurofibromatoses: A Pathogenic and Clinical Overview. London:
                  Chapman and Hall Medical.
Huson, S. M., and M. Upadhyaya
   1994   Neurofibromatosis 1: Clinical Management and Genetic Counselling. *In*
                  The Neurofibromatoses: A Pathogenic and Clinical Overview. S. M. Huson
                  and R.A.C. Hughes, eds. Pp. 355–382. London: Chapman and Hall Medi-
                  cal.
Hyden, Lars-Christer
   1995   The Rhetoric of Recovery and Change. Culture, Medicine and Psychiatry
                  19:73–90.
Ingstad, Benedicte, and Susan Reynolds Whyte
   1995   Disability and Culture. Berkeley: University of California Press.
Jonsen, Albert R.
   1996   The Impact of Mapping the Human Genome on the Patient-Physician
                  Relationship. *In* the Human Genome Project and the Future of Health Care.
                  Thomas H. Murray, Mark A. Rothstein, and Robert F. Murry, Jr., eds. Pp.
                  1–20. Bloomington and Indianapolis, IN: Indiana University Press.
Kessler, S.
   1984   Psychologic Responses to Stresses in Genetic Disease. *In* Genetic Disor-
                  ders and Birth Defects in Families and Society: Toward Interdisciplinary
                  Understanding. Pp. 114–117. White Plains, NY: March of Dimes Birth
                  Defects Foundation.
Kleinman, Arthur
   1988   The Illness Narratives: Suffering, Healing, and the Human Condition. New
                  York: Basic Books.
Korf, Bruce R.
   1988   The Neurofibromatoses: What Do We Know about Them? Postgraduate
                  Medicine 83(2):79–85.
   1990   Diagnosis of Neurofibromatosis and Clinical Overview. *In* Neurofibroma-
                  tosis: A Handbook for Patients, Families, and Health Care Professionals.
                  A. Rubenstein and B. Korf, eds. Pp. 15–28. New York: Thieme Medical
                  Publishers Inc.
Kubler-Ross, E.
   1969   On Death and Dying. New York: Macmillan.
Lansdown, R., J. Lloyd, and J. Hunter
   1991   Facial Deformity in Childhood: Severity and Psychological Adjustment.
                  Child Care, Health and Development 17:165–171.

LaPlante, Mitchell P.
1992   How Many Americans Have a Disability? Disability Statistics Abstract, No. 5, December. Disability Statistics Program, University of California, San Francisco.

Lewandowski, Lawrence, and Karen Arcangelo
1994   The Social Adjustment and Self-Concept of Adults with Learning Disabilities. Journal of Learning Disabilities 27(9):598–605.

Listernick, R., M. J. Greenwald, and N. A. Easterly
1989   Optic Gliomas in Children with Neurofibromatosis Type 1. Journal of Pediatrics 114:788–792.

Livneh, H. A.
1988   A Dimensional Perspective on the Origin of Negative Attitudes Toward Persons with Disabilities. In Attitudes Toward Persons with Disabilities. H. Yuker, ed. Pp. 35–46. New York: Springer Publishing Company.

Longmore, Paul
1985   Screening Stereotypes: Images of Disabled People. Social Policy 16(1)2:31–37.

Marchac, D.
1984   Intracranial Enlargement of the Orbital Cavity and Palpebral Remodeling for Orbto Palpebral Orbitopalpebral Neurofibromatosis. Plastic and Reconstructive Surgery 73(4):534–541.

McCulloh, Craig
1998   Limb Lengthening: A Cure to Dwarfism? Little People of America Newsletter. LPA Today 35(3):14.

Messner, Roberta L.
1986   Gastrointestinal Considerations in Neurofibromatosis. Society of Gastrointestinal Assistants Journal (Summer):3–8.

Messner, Roberta L., Sylvia Gardner, and Mark R. Messner
1985   Neurofibromatosis—an International Enigma: A Framework for Nursing. Cancer Nursing 8(6):314–322.

Messner, Roberta L., Messner, Mark R., and Susan J. Lewis
1985   Neurofibromatosis: A Familial and Family Disorder. Journal of Neurosurgical Nursing 17(4):221–228.

Messner, Roberta L., and Martha Neff Smith
1986   Neurofibromatosis: Relinquishing the Masks; A Quest for Quality of Life. Journal of Advanced Nursing 11:459–464.

Miller, H. H., L. J. Bauman, D. R. Friedman, and J. J. De Cosse
1986–1987   Psychosocial Adjustment of Familial Polyposis Patients and Participation in Chemoprevention Trials. International Journal of Psychiatry in Medicine 16(3):211–230.

Miller, M., and J. G. Hall
1978   Possible Maternal Effect on Severity of Neurofibromatosis. Lancet 2:1071–1072.

Montagu, Ashley
1971   The Elephant Man: A Study in Human Dignity. New York: Outerbridge and Dienstfrey. Distributed by E. P. Dutton.
1979   The Elephant Man: A Study in Human Dignity. Second Edition. New York: E. P. Dutton.

Mouridsen, Svend Erik, and Sven Asger Sorensen
 1995   Psychological Aspects of von Recklinghausen Neurofibromatosis (NF1).
                   Medical Genetics (32):921–924.
Mulvihill, John H.
 1990   Introduction and History. *In* Neurofibromatosis: A Handbook for Patients,
                   Families, and Health Care Professionals. A.E. Rubenstein and B.R. Korf,
                   eds. Pp. 1–12. New York: Thieme Medical Publishers Inc.
Murphy, Robert
 1990   The Body Silent. New York: W. W. Norton.
Murray, Thomas H., Mark A. Rothstein, and Robert F. Murry, Jr., eds.
 1996   The Human Genome Project and the Future of Health Care. Bloomington
                   and Indianapolis, IN: Indiana University Press.
Myerson, Loreen
 1995   Empathetic Versus Clinical Encounters with Ehlers-Danlos Syndrome.
                   Anthropology of Work Review 15 (2–3):22–27.
Nachtigall, R. D., G. Becker, and M. Wozny
 1992   The Effects of Gender-Specific Diagnosis on Men's and Women's Re-
                   sponse to Infertility. Fertility Sterility 57:113–121.
National Institutes of Health
 1988   Neurofibromatosis. National Institutes of Health Consensus Development
                   Conference Statement. Archives of Neurology 45:575–578.
The National Neurofibromatosis Foundation, Inc.
 1988   Childhood Learning Disabilities in Neurofibromatosis, Conference Series
                   Volume 1. New York.
Nester, Anne
 1997   Pre-Employment Testing and the ADA. Program on Employment and
                   Disability. New York: Cornell University Press.
Neurofibromatosis, Inc.
 1991   Reprint of NIH Concensus Development Conference Statement. Update
                   Four Years Later by John J. Mulvihill. Mitchellville, MD: Neurofibroma-
                   tosis, Inc.
Newsweek
 1988   What the Elephant Man Really Had. 29 February.
North, K. N., V. Riccardi, C. Samango-Sprouse, R. Ferner, B. Moore, E. Legius, N. Ratner,
and M. B. Denckla
 1997   Cognitive Function and Academic Performance in Neurofibromatosis 1:
                   Consensus Statement from the NF1 Cognitive Disorders Task Force. Neu-
                   rology 48:1121–1127.
Quaid, Kimberly A.
 1994   A Few Words from a "Wise" Woman. *In* Genes and Human Self-Knowl-
                   edge. Robert F. Weir, Susan C. Lawrence, and Evan Fales, eds. Pp. 3–17.
                   Iowa City: University of Iowa Press.
Riccardi, Vincent M.
 1992   Neurofibromatosis: Phenotype, Natural History, and Pathogenesis. Balti-
                   more: The Johns Hopkins University Press.
 1996   Educating Clinicians about Genetics. *In* The Human Genome Project and
                   the Future of Health Care. Thomas H. Murray, Mark A. Rothstein, and

Robert F. Murry, Jr., eds. Pp. 21–38. Bloomington and Indianapolis, IN: Indiana University Press.

Richman, L., and D. Harper
1978   School Adjustment of Children with Observable Disabilities. Journal of Abnormal Psychology 6:11–18.

Robinson, Ian
1990   Personal Narratives, Social Careers, and Medical Courses: Analyzing Life Trajectories in Autobiography of People with Multiple Sclerosis. Social Science and Medicine 30(11):1173–1186.

Rubenstein, A., and B. Korf, eds.
1990   Neurofibromatosis: A Handbook for Patients, Families, and Health-Care Professionals. New York: Thieme Medical Publishers Inc.

Safilios-Rothschild, C.
1977   Societal Reactions to Disability. *In* Social and Psychological Aspects of Disability. J. Stubbins, ed. Baltimore: University Park Press.

Scheer, Jessica, and Nora Groce
1988   Impairment as a Human Constant: Cross-Cultural and Historical Perspectives on Variation. Journal of Social Issues 44(1):23–37.

Scotch, Richard K.
1988   Disability as a Basis for Social Movement: Advocacy and the Politics of Definition. Journal of Social Issues 44(1):159–172.

Seward, G. R.
1994   Did the Elephant Man Have Neurofibromatosis 1? *In* The Neurofibromatoses: A Pathogenic and Clinical Overview. S. M. Huson and R.A.C. Hughes, eds. Pp. 382–401. London: Chapman and Hall Medical.

Sitlington, Patricia L., Alan R. Frank, and Rori Carson
1992   Adult Adjustment among High School Graduates with Mild Disabilities. Exceptional Children 59(3):221–233.

Solomon, Lawrence M.
1968   Quasimodo's Diagnosis. Journal of the American Medical Association 204: 190–191.

Suzuki, David, and Peter Knudtson
1990   Genethics: The Clash between the New Genetics and Human Values. Second Edition. Cambridge, MA: Harvard University Press.

Tibbles, J., and M. Cohen
1986   Proteus Syndrome: The Elephant Man Diagnosed. British Medical Journal 293:683–685.

Time
1979   29 January.

Treves, Frederick
1885   A Case of Congenital Deformity. The Transactions of the Pathological Society of London 36:494–498.
1923   The Elephant Man and Other Reminiscences. London: Cassell.

Trevisani, Thomas P., Alan L. Pohl, and Hani S. Matloub
1982   Neurofibroma of the Ear: Function and Aesthetics. Plastic and Reconstructive Surgery 70(2):217–219.

United States Equal Employment Opportunity Commission
   1991   The Americans with Disabilities Act: Your Responsibilities as Employer.
                 Washington, DC.
Upadhyaya, M., and D. N. Cooper
   1998   Neurofibromatosis Type 1: From Genotype to Phenotype. Herndon, VA:
                 BIOS Scientific Publishers.
Variety
   1979   7 March.
Ventimiglia, C., and P. Balestrazzi
   1996   *Famiglie con NF1 Percorsi socio-sanitari, nodi problematici del vivere
                 quotidiano e reti di sostegno.* Istituto di Sociologia e di Clinica Pediartica
                 Universita delgi Studi di Parma. Via Gramsci, 14–43100 Parma: Associaz-
                 ione NeuroFibromatosi.
von Recklinghausen, Friedrich
   1882   *Ueber die Multiplen Fibrome der Haut und ihre Beziehung zu den Multiplen
                 Neuromen.* Berlin: A. Hirschwald.
Wallander, J., J. Varni, L. Babani, H. Banis, and T. Wilcox
   1989   Family Resources as Resistance Factors for Psychological Maladjustment
                 in Chronically Ill and Handicapped Children. Journal of Pediatric Psychol-
                 ogy 14:157–173.
Weir, Robert F., Susan C. Lawrence, and Evan Fales, eds.
   1994   Genes and Human Self-Knowledge: Historical and Philosophical Reflec-
                 tions on Modern Genetics. Iowa City: University of Iowa Press.
Weiss, Joan O., and Jayne S. Mackta
   1996   Starting and Sustaining Genetic Support Groups. Baltimore: The Johns
                 Hopkins University Press.
Wellman, Barbara
   1990   Impact of Neurofibromatosis on the Adolescent. *In* Neurofibromatosis: A
                 Handbook for Patients, Families, and Health Care Professionals. A. Ruben-
                 stein and B. Korf, eds. Pp. 211–215. New York: Thieme Medical Publishers
                 Inc.
Whyte, Susan Reynolds, and Benedicte Ingstad
   1995   Disability and Culture: An Overview. *In* Disability and Culture. B. Ingstad
                 and S. R. Whyte, eds. Pp. 3–32. Berkeley: University of California Press.
Wilson, Mary Ann, and Felice Yahr
   1990   Impact of Neurofibromatosis on the Family. *In* Neurofibromatosis: A
                 Handbook for Patients, Families, and Health Care Professionals. A. Ruben-
                 stein and B. Korf, eds. Pp. 216–224. New York: Thieme Medical Publishers
                 Inc.
Wynbrandt, James, and Mark D. Ludman
   1991   The Encyclopedia of Genetic Disorders and Birth Defects. New York and
                 Oxford: Facts on File.
Yuker, H., ed.
   1988   Attitudes Toward Persons with Disabilities. Albany, NY: Springer Publish-
                 ing Company.
Zanca, A., and A. Zanka
   1980   Antique Illustrations of Neurofibromatosis. International Journal of Der-
                 matology 19:55–58.

Zola, Kenneth
   1985   Depictions of Disability—Metaphor, Message and Medium in the Media:
                 A Research and Political Agenda. Social Science Journal 22:5–17.

Index

About the Author

JOAN ABLON is Professor Emerita, Medical Anthropology Program, Department of Anthropology, History, and Social Medicine, School of Medicine, University of California, San Francisco. She is the author of *Little People in America* (Praeger, 1984) and *Living with Difference* (Praeger, 1988).